OXFORD DIABETES LIBRARY

Diabetic Retinopathy: screening to treatment

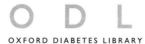

O D L

OXFORD DIABETES LIBRARY

Diabetic Retinopathy: screening to treatment

Edited by

Professor Paul M. Dodson

Aston University, Birmingham, UK and
Consultant in Diabetes and Ophthalmic Medicine,
Departments of Diabetes, Ophthalmology and Heart
of England Diabetic Retinopathy Screening Centre,
Birmingham, UK

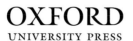

OXFORD
UNIVERSITY PRESS

OXFORD

UNIVERSITY PRESS

Great Clarendon Street, Oxford OX2 6DP

Oxford University Press is a department of the University of Oxford.
It furthers the University's objective of excellence in research, scholarship,
and education by publishing worldwide in

Oxford New York

Auckland Cape Town Dar es Salaam Hong Kong Karachi
Kuala Lumpur Madrid Melbourne Mexico City Nairobi
New Delhi Shanghai Taipei Toronto

With offices in

Argentina Austria Brazil Chile Czech Republic France Greece
Guatemala Hungary Italy Japan Poland Portugal Singapore
South Korea Switzerland Thailand Turkey Ukraine Vietnam

Oxford is a registered trade mark of Oxford University Press
in the UK and in certain other countries

Published in the United States
by Oxford University Press Inc., New York

© Oxford University Press, 2008

The moral rights of the authors have been asserted
Database right Oxford University Press (maker)

First published 2008
Reprinted 2009

British Library Cataloguing in Publication Data

Data available

Library of Congress Cataloging in Publication Data

Data available

Typeset by Newgen Imaging Systems (P) Ltd., Chennai, India
Printed in Great Britain
on acid-free paper by
Ashford Colour Press Ltd., Gosport, Hampshire

ISBN 978-0-19-954496-7

10 9 8 7 6 5 4 3 2

Contents

Preface *vii*

Contributors *ix*

Symbols and abbreviations *xi*

1 What is diabetes?
Alexander Wright
1

2 Diabetic retinopathy—reasons
for screening
Margaret Clarke
11

3 Anatomy of the eye and the healthy fundus
Laurence Quant
17

4 Diabetes and the eye
Paul M Dodson
33

5 Background diabetic retinopathy
Laurence Quant
45

6 Maculopathy
Rebecca Lone
49

7 Pre-proliferative and proliferative retinopathy
Rebecca Leigh
59

8 Advanced diabetic eye disease
Karen Whitehouse
71

9 Other ophthalmic lesions in the fundus
Jonathan M Gibson
79

10 The screening episode—visual acuity,
    mydriasis, and digital photography
    David Roy and Jane Pitt   9

11 How to Grade
    Helen C King   10

12 The principles of a national diabetic
    retinopathy screening programme
    Margaret Clarke   11

13 Programme administration
    Helen C King and Caroline Harrison   12

14 Models of screening and IT
    Andrew Mills   13

15 Training and accreditation for retinal screening
    Margaret Clarke   14

16 Medical management of diabetic retinopathy
    Paul M Dodson   15

17 Ophthalmic treatment of diabetic retinopathy
    Jonathan M Gibson   16

    Appendix: Screening intervals, other DR grading
    systems and visual acuity scales   17

    Index *177*

Preface

As the epidemic of diabetes unfolds, the need for additional treatments and amelioration of diabetic complications becomes ever more pressing. Whilst research continues into new therapies, the feared complications of diabetes are still too common across the world, with blindness the number one to many patients.

Laser treatment has been the mainstay of delaying and preventing visual loss, but needs to be given at an early stage for best effect. This has led to the concept of screening to pick up diabetic retinopathy (DR) at an early asymptomatic stage, and hence maximize treatment benefit.

The UK is currently embarking on a diabetic retinopathy screening programme using digital technology, encompassing the four nations of Wales, Scotland, Northern Ireland, and England (www.retinalscreening.co.uk), comparable to the cervical and breast cancer screening programmes already in place. To achieve this has required considerable investment in both capital equipment and recruitment of new staff, including photographers, screeners, graders, optometrists, nurses, administrators, commissioners, and clinicians in diabetes and ophthalmology.

This pocketbook aims to be a concise companion for those professionals involved in the diabetic retinopathy screening programme and contains the important principles of screening and outlines the basis of current protocols which are evolving as the DR screening programme progresses. It gives the basis of many of the competencies of the Certificate of Diabetic Retinopathy Screening (City and Guilds, London) qualification required for accreditation of screening personnel. The pocket size of this book does not allow an exhaustive description of every aspect of diabetic retinopathy or the differences between the four nations' screening programmes. It is a summary of the basis of screening and practical information, with no intention of diminishing the important variations in schemes, for example, in grading levels, numbers of photographs taken per eye, and the use of mydriasis. It also includes some additional features of our own Birmingham scheme (www.retinopathyscreening.co.uk).

The book covers the basics of diabetes mellitus and ocular anatomy for those new to the subject, leading onto why screening is required, and the epidemiology and nature of diabetic retinopathy and associated ocular diseases. It includes descriptions of the principles of screening, grading, and administration, with the final sections on the modern treatment of diabetic retinopathy from both a medical and an ophthalmology perspective. A section is included on the important area of information technology which underpins computers, digital imaging, connectivity, and servers, and an appendix summarizing screening intervals, grading schemes and comparative visual acuity scales. Each chapter has some further reading references and sources of information including websites, with the English DR screening workbook providing an invaluable reference (www.retinalscreening.co.uk).

I am very grateful to my Consultant colleagues (Prof. Jonathan Gibson, Dr Margaret Clarke and Dr Alexander Wright) and all the contributors to the book who are part of the Birmingham and Black Country Diabetic Retinopathy Screening Programme.

I must thank all those at Oxford University Press for making this book possible, to Andrew Mills and Helen King for editorial assistance, and my wife Lynne, and family (James, Alex and Ellie) for their continual support.

Paul Dodson

Contributors

Margaret Clarke
Consultant Physician
Heartlands NHS Foundation
Trust, Birmingham, UK

Jonathan M Gibson
Professor of Ophthalmology
University of Aston,
Birmingham, UK

Caroline Harrison
Screening Programme Manager
Heart of England Diabetic
Retinopathy Screening Centre,
Birmingham, UK

Helen C King
Retinal Screener
Heart of England Diabetic
Retinopathy Screening Centre,
Birmingham, UK

Rebecca Leigh
Retinal Screener
Heart of England Diabetic
Retinopathy Screening Centre,
Birmingham, UK

Rebecca Lone
Retinal Screener
Heart of England Diabetic
Retinopathy Screening Centre,
Birmingham, UK

Andrew Mills
IT Consultant
Heart of England Diabetic
Retinopathy Screening Centre,
Birmingham, UK

Jane Pitt
Retinal Screener and
Head of Training
Heart of England Diabetic
Retinopathy Screening Centre,
Birmingham, UK

Laurence Quant
Retinal Screener
Heart of England Diabetic
Retinopathy Screening Centre,
Birmingham, UK

David Roy
Principal Retinal Screener
Heart of England Diabetic
Retinopathy Screening Centre,
Birmingham, UK

Karen Whitehouse
Retinal Screener
Heart of England Diabetic
Retinopathy Screening Centre,
Birmingham, UK

A Wright
Consultant Physician
Heartlands NHS Foundation
Trust, Birmingham, UK

Symbols and abbreviations

AC	anterior chamber
ACE	angiotensin converting enzyme
AGE	advanced glycation end product
AMD	age-related macular degeneration
APEL	acquired prior experiential learning
ARB	angiotensin receptor blockers
BP	blood pressure
BRVO	branch retinal vein occlusion
CARDS	Collaborative Atorvastatin Diabetes Study
CHRPE	congenital hypertrophy of the retinal pigment epithelium
CPU	central processing unit
CRVO	central retinal vein occlusion
CSII	continuous subcutaneous infusion of short-acting insulin
CSMO	clinically significant macula oedema
CV	cardiovascular
2D	2 dimensional
3D	3 dimensional
2DD	2 disc diameters
DCCT	Diabetes Control and Complications Trial
DIRECT	Diabetic Retinopathy Candesartan Trial
DR	diabetic retinopathy
DRS2	Diabetic Retinopathy Study
ECG	electrocadiogram
ERM	epi-retinal membrane
ESR	erythrocyte sedimentation rate
ETDRS	Early Treatment Diabetic Retinopathy Study
EUCLID	EURODIAB Controlled Trial of Lisinopril in Insulin-Dependent Diabetes
FDA	Food and Drugs Administration
FFA	fluorescein angiography
FGF	fibroblast growth factor

FIELD	Fenofibrate Intervention and Event Lowering in Diabetes
GFR	glomerula filtration rate
GH	growth hormone
GPs	general practitioners
HbA1c	glycated haemoglobin
HD	hard disc
HDL	high density lipoprotein
HES	hospital eye service
IGF	insulin growth factor
IRMAs	intra-retinal microvascular abnormalities
IT	information technology
JPEG	joint photographic experts group
JPG	joint photographic group
LDL-C	low-density lipoprotein-cholesterol
M	maculopathy grade
NHS	National Health Service
NLH	notional learning hours
NPL	no perception of light
NSC	National Screening Committee
NSF	National Service Framework
NVD	new vessels of the optic disc
NVE	new vessels elsewhere
OCT	optical coherence tomography
OS	operating system
PCT	Primary Care Trust
PDR	proliferative diabetic retinopathy
PGD	patient group directive
PKC	protein kinase C
PL	perception of light
POAG	primary open angle glaucoma
PRP	pan-retinal photocoagulation
QA	quality assurance
R	retinopathy grade
RAM	random access memory
RPE	retinal pigment epithelium

RVO	retinal vein occlusion
SVI	severe visual impairment
TZD	thiazolidinedione
U	ungradable
UKPDS	United Kingdom Prospective Diabetes Study
USB	universal serial bus
VA	visual acuity
VEGF	vascular endothelial growth factor
VI	visual impairment
VPNs	visual private networks
VRQ	vocationally related qualification
WHO	World Health Organisation

Chapter 1

What is diabetes?

Alexander Wright

> **Key points**
>
> - Diabetes mellitus is characterized by raised levels of glucose in the blood. This may result in symptoms of excessive thirst, passing of more urine, loss of weight and loss of energy, and eventually, damage to a number of tissues.
> - At present diabetes is classified into type 1, type 2, secondary, and those due to other less common causes.
> - Acute complications occur when plasma glucose levels fall below normal ('hypoglycaemia') or are very high with resulting loss of fluid and development of ketones.
> - Chronic complications may arise with long-term damage to blood vessels, nerves, kidneys, retina, and the lens.
> - Good control of glucose levels and good management of other vascular 'risk factors' can maintain health and prevent or delay long-term complications.

1.1 What is diabetes mellitus?

Diabetes mellitus is a disorder of sugar metabolism caused by insufficient action of insulin. The basic sugar in the body is glucose, and energy comes from the metabolism of glucose in all cells. Energy is needed to keep every cell of the body in good health. The brain and nervous tissue are dependent on glucose as their only source of fuel. Glucose is an active molecule and the body has tight control mechanisms in place to keep the amount of glucose in the blood as steady as possible. Reserves of glucose are stored as glycogen in the liver and muscles so, when starving, glucose can be added to the blood stream to stop levels from falling below a critical concentration of about 4mmol/L.

Glucose is mobilized from stores with the help of hormones such as adrenaline, glucagon, and cortisol. Ultimately, we depend on a regular intake of food containing sugars to keep going. A few of the sugars we eat are simple ones such as glucose, sucrose (table sugar), fructose, maltose, and lactose in milk, but most of the sugars we eat are complex sugars known as carbohydrates, mostly starch. On digestion in the gut, carbohydrates are turned into simple sugars such as glucose. After glucose enters the blood stream from the gut following a meal it is taken into tissues. Glucose gets into some tissues such as the brain quite freely but cannot get into muscle and fat without the help of insulin. Insulin is therefore important to stop blood levels of glucose from going too high, the upper limit in a normal person being set at about 6mmol/L fasting and about 11mmol/L after food. Diabetes occurs when these levels are exceeded—for the precise definitions see Section 1.1.1. High glucose levels are the most obvious effect of insufficient insulin action (see Figure 1.1).

The fundamental defect causing diabetes is lack of insulin action. Insulin is a small protein made in groups of cells, known as beta cells, in the islets of Langerhans within the pancreas. A small amount of basal insulin is secreted all the time to keep glucose stores under control, but a much larger amount is secreted as soon as food is ingested to help dispose of the glucose load. Insufficient insulin action arises either because the islets are damaged and do not make enough insulin (insulin deficiency), or because insulin is produced but cannot work properly because of build-up of resistance to the action of insulin in fat and muscle (insulin resistance), the latter commonly associated with obesity.

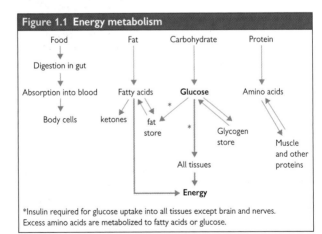

Figure 1.1 Energy metabolism

*Insulin required for glucose uptake into all tissues except brain and nerves.
Excess amino acids are metabolized to fatty acids or glucose.

1.1.1 **Definition**

Diabetes is defined by the World Health Organisation (WHO) as a fasting venous plasma glucose concentration of equal to or greater than 7.0mmol/L or a venous plasma glucose concentration of equal or greater than 11.1mmol/L 2 hours after taking 75g glucose by mouth. It should be appreciated that in the general population plasma glucose concentrations are a continuous variable and there is no natural cut-off based on glucose criteria alone to say when diabetes starts. The glucose levels used to define diabetes have been chosen from studying large populations and noting the glucose level at which diabetic retinopathy (DR) develops—that is, it is above these concentrations that the risk of retinopathy becomes measurable. There are categories of lesser degrees of glucose intolerance which are of relevance to vascular disease, metabolic syndrome, and gestational diabetes, but as these are not risk factors for retinopathy, such patients do not qualify for retinal screening. The diagnostic pathway for diabetes is shown in Box 1.1.

A glucose tolerance test using a 75g glucose intake is performed if the diagnosis is not established by the random or fasting blood glucose values as described in Box 1.1. The diagnostic criteria are shown in Box 1.2, and also illustrate the values diagnostic of impaired fasting glycaemia and impaired glucose intolerance.

Box 1.1 Diagnostic pathway of diabetes mellitus

Think of the diagnosis if

Excessive thirst and passing of urine, weight loss, tiredness, incontinence, vulval or penile rash, foot ulcer, blurred vision

Suspect diagnosis if

Urine positive for glucose

Confirm diagnosis by

Measuring glucose level in blood
Test urine for ketones if positive for glucose

Diabetes diagnosed if

Symptoms plus blood glucose > 7.0 fasting
or 11.1mmol/L post meal **or**
no symptoms and blood glucose abnormal on two separate occasions.

(Consider the diagnosis of type 1 diabetes if abnormal blood glucose *and* moderate or heavy ketonuria. Sometimes anti-islet cell antibodies are measured to confirm the autoimmune process. Consider the diagnosis of type 2 diabetes if abnormal blood glucose *but* no or light ketonuria.)

Box 1.2 Definition of different degrees of glucose intolerance		
	Venous plasma glucose (mmol/L)	
	Overnight fast	2 hours post-glucose load
Diabetes mellitus	≥7.0	and/or ≥11.1
Impaired glucose tolerance	<7.0	and ≥7.8–<11.1
Impaired fasting glycaemia	≥6.0 to <7.0	and if measured <7.8

1.2 Classification of diabetes

Diabetes is a syndrome that has many causes and varies widely in symptoms from the asymptomatic to the acutely ill. The current classification of diabetes (WHO 1980) is largely based on clinical criteria and uses knowledge of the cause only to a limited extent. The basic subdivision is into type 1, type 2, and other causes of diabetes. Most diabetes tends to run in families and is slightly more common in men than in women.

1.2.1 Type 1 diabetes

Type 1 diabetes results from a total lack of insulin caused by destruction of the islets of Langerhans in the pancreas by an autoimmune process occurring in genetically susceptible people. It can occur at any age, but onset is usually before the age of 30. The trigger or triggers for the autoimmune process have not been identified. In type 1 diabetes occurring in older people, the autoimmune process tends to be slower than in children. Type 1 diabetes occurs in approximately 1/250 of the population of the United Kingdom and is relatively rare in some ethnic groups such as Afro-Caribbeans, Chinese, and Japanese. The disease process occurs over 2 to 3 years, but tends to present clinically with rather sudden onset. Treatment is always by insulin, usually starting as soon as the diagnosis is made, and insulin is essential for life.

1.2.2 Type 2 diabetes

Type 2 diabetes is a more common condition occurring with increasing frequency, and is now present in approximately 5% of the UK population. Some racial groups have higher prevalence, particularly those of Asian origin, the most extreme being the Pima Indians of Arizona. Type 2 diabetes is a more complex problem having resistance to the action of insulin and also failure of insulin production. There are probably many different subtypes which, at present, are conveniently grouped together under the same diagnosis. The usual patient with type 2 diabetes is a middle-aged or elderly subject, overweight, and with a family history of diabetes. Insulin resistance is probably the initiating factor followed by a gradual loss of insulin secretion, occurring over many years. In the initial stages, treatment of type 2 diabetes is often dietary together with modifiers of insulin sensitivity, followed by attempts to stimulate insulin secretion. It is only some years later that insulin replacement therapy is needed.

Other causes of type 2 diabetes include single gene defects, and various inherited syndromes (e.g. mitochondrial diabetes). Secondary diabetes may occur resulting from damage to the pancreas (i.e. affecting insulin secretion) such as pancreatitis, iron deposition, cystic fibrosis, surgical removal of the pancreas, or drugs and hormones that increase insulin resistance (for example, steroid therapy) and excess amounts of cortisol, growth hormone, and glucagon.

1.3 **Complications of diabetes**

Glucose can damage tissues by altering proteins—the so-called browning effect. One of the proteins altered by glucose is haemoglobin, and this change is utilized in the monitoring of diabetes by measurements of glycated haemoglobin (HbA1c)—that is, how much glucose has become attached to the protein haemoglobin in the red cells and expressed as a percentage of total haemoglobin. This allows an average measurement of blood glucose control over a 6- to 8-week period.

The complications are divided into two broad categories, macro- and microvascular, and are listed in Box 1.3.

Box 1.3 Complications of diabetes

Macrovascular (large vessel)
- Coronary: angina, heart attacks, heart failure
- Carotid and cerebral: stroke, disturbance of vision
- Peripheral: pain on walking, foot ulceration, gangrene.

Microvascular (small vessel)
- Eye: retinopathy, cataract, glaucoma
- Kidney (nephropathy): leaking of albumin in the urine, nephrotic syndrome, renal failure
- Nervous system (neuropathy): peripheral nerve damage, muscle wasting, cranial nerve palsies, autonomic nerve damage
- Skin: fungal infections, carbuncles and pyoderma gangrenosum, necrobiosis
- Joints: stiffness of the fingers, Charcot foot, frozen shoulder.

1.3.1 **Macrovascular disease**

The brunt of tissue damage by glucose falls on the blood vessels. Premature atherosclerosis leads to large-vessel disease (macrovascular disease), which results in stroke (cerebrovascular disease) and heart attack (myocardial infarction) that occur 2–3 times more commonly in diabetes. This may also reduce the blood supply to the lower limbs (peripheral vascular disease), leading to pain on walking (intermittent claudication), skin ulceration, and ultimately lower limb amputation. The arterial circulation to the kidneys may be reduced (renal artery stenosis), which may accelerate kidney failure. Because of the devastating effects of macrovascular disease in diabetic subjects, some clinicians have offered an alternative definition of the reality of diabetes mellitus:

> A state of premature cardiovascular death associated with hyperglycaemia, and may be with blindness, renal failure, and lower limb amputation.

1.3.2 **Microvascular disease**

The effect of glucose damaging the smaller blood vessels (microvascular disease) is seen in the eye with retinopathy and in the kidneys with renal failure (DR), and contributes to damage of the peripheral nerves with neuropathy. There are also effects of glucose on the lens causing cataracts and to some extent in the skin and in the hand causing thickening of soft tissues, due to excess glycosylation of collagen.

The degree of damage by glucose is related to both the level of blood glucose control, that is, overall blood glucose control, and to the duration of diabetes. The long-term complications of diabetes are rarely found in the first 5 to 10 years of diabetes but increasingly thereafter.

This means that in type 1 diabetes, complications are not seen during the first 5 to 10 years after diagnosis but in type 2 diabetes with a much slower, insidious onset, complications may be present at the time of diagnosis. These findings are crucial as to when retinopathy screening begins in diabetic patients:

> Type 1—first retinal screen after 5 to 8 years of disease duration before 12 years of age and annually in all patients subsequently.

> Type 2—first screen at diagnosis of diabetes and annually thereafter.

Complications, however, are not inevitable because good blood glucose and blood pressure control can prevent or delay their onset.

1.4 **Principles of treatment**

Overall control of diabetes greatly affects not only the general well-being of the patient with diabetes but also the outcome of diabetes-related complications. Beneficial effects of blood glucose control have been shown with significant reductions, in particular of microvascular problems, in both type 1 diabetes (DCCT (Diabetes Control and Complications Trial) studies) and type 2 diabetes (United Kingdom Prospective Diabetes Study (UKPDS)). Of importance is the finding that any improvement of glucose control is of benefit and that there is no threshold effect.

To achieve optimal glucose control requires a motivated patient having initial and then updated education, working with a multi-professional team including the general practitioner, diabetes specialist nurse, dietitian, podiatrist, and where necessary the specialist care team. Structured care, including regular check-ups on glucose control, blood pressure, lipids, and the health of the feet and eyes are important aspects of diabetes management that affect outcome.

For type 1 diabetes insulin therapy is started immediately and is continued for life. Insulin techniques with a syringe, continuous infusion pump, or injector pen need to be taught and understood. Advice on diet, counting carbohydrates, and life style, monitoring of blood glucose concentrations, and avoidance of low-blood glucose attacks (hypoglycaemia) are all part of the education. Moderating alcohol and not smoking are also important. The price of tight blood glucose control in type 1 patients is multiple attendances, regular home blood glucose monitoring, weight gain, and risk of hypoglycaemia. The latter problem has consequences for driving and employment.

In type 2 diabetes the first approach is dietary, often with advice on reducing the intake of simple sugars and calories, if overweight, and increasing the amount of exercise where possible. Alcohol consumption should be moderated and information given on smoking cessation. This initial advice is often combined with attempts to reduce insulin resistance with metformin or a glitazone. Special efforts to encourage weight loss may be used, including drugs such as orlistat and rimonabant. When these methods fail to control blood glucose levels, drugs that stimulate the beta cells to produce more insulin are used. The common groups are the sulfonylureas and metiglinides. More recently, therapy with incretins has been shown to be effective either alone or in combination with other drugs. After a period of time that is rather variable, but commonly between 5 and 10 years, oral therapy ceases to be adequate and insulin therapy is started as in a patient with type 1 diabetes. The principles of management are shown in Table 1.1 and Figure 1.2.

Table 1.1 Basic management of diabetes

Diet and life style
- Improving insulin sensitivity—metformin or thiazolidinediones
- Stimulating insulin secretion sulfonylureas, metiglinides, incretins

Replacement insulin
- Subcutaneous injections (1–5 times a day depending on the type of insulin); short-acting insulin to cover meals long-acting insulin to cover basal needs
- Continuous subcutaneous infusion of short-acting insulin (CSII)

(Commonly used insulins are short-acting: Actrapid®, Apidra®, Humalog® given three times daily. Long-acting: Detemir®, Glargine®, Isophane® given once or twice daily. Mixtures of short-acting and Isophane® insulin (30/70% or 50/50%) given twice or three times daily)

Figure 1.2 Management principles of type 2 diabetes

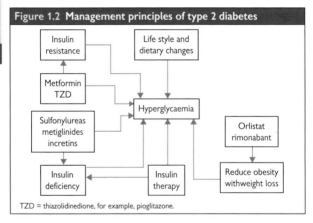

TZD = thiazolidinedione, for example, pioglitazone.

Diabetes mellitus is a disease that is increasing in prevalence across the Western world in epidemic proportions. It has potentially devastating consequences to health, owing to hyperglycaemic symptoms and adverse effects on both macro- and microvascular disease. Although better outcomes can be achieved with effective medical management and patient compliance, none of the modern hypoglycaemic therapies have a specific targeted effect on microvascular disease, but rely on the beneficial effect of optimal glycaemic control. Modern medical management for macrovascular disease is with optimal treatment of cardiovascular risk factors with anti-hypertensive agents, statins, and aspirin therapy.

Further reading

Fox C and Kilvert A (2007). *Type 1 diabetes at your fingertips*. Class Publishing, London.

Fox C and Kilvert A (2008). Type 2 *diabetes at your fingertips*. Class Publishing, London.

Krentz AJ and Bailey CJ (2005). *Type 2 diabetes in practice*. Royal Society of Medicine Press, London 2nd edition.

Williams G and Pickup J (2004). *The handbook of diabetes*. Blackwell Publishing, Oxford.

Chapter 2

Diabetic retinopathy— reasons for screening

Margaret Clarke

Key points

- Diabetic retinopathy (DR) is still one of the commonest causes of visual loss in the Western world in the working age population.
- Patients with visual loss due to DR often reflect late presentation or non-attendance to diabetes and eye services.
- The pattern of blindness in diabetes is that maculopathy is the major cause, particularly in type 2 diabetic subjects, whereas blindness due to proliferative retinopathy is becoming rarer in type 1 diabetes.
- DR meets the screening criteria of Wilson and Jungner for a successful programme; as it has important adverse effects, laser treatment is effective, it can be easily detected by digital photography, which is an acceptable test, and is cost-effective.

2.1 Introduction

Diabetic retinopathy (DR) is a microangiopathy affecting the retinal vasculature, leading to progressive retinal damage that may end in complete visual loss and blindness (see definition in end of Chapter Appendix). DR still remains one of the commonest causes of blindness worldwide.

Despite advances in diabetes care and laser photocoagulation of the retina, visual loss is still all too common for the following reasons:

- Late presentation for treatment (it is often well advanced before symptoms develop)
- Non-attendance at diabetic services
- Lack of response in some cases of maculopathy and proliferative retinopathy to laser treatment.

2.2 **Causes of visual loss in diabetic subjects**

DR is the biggest single cause of blindness in the UK population of working-age people. Studies have shown that approximately 10% of diabetic subjects will have DR requiring diabetic eye clinic care. Without treatment, 6–9% of patients with proliferative retinopathy will become blind and 10% of patients with diabetic maculopathy develop moderate visual loss annually. A recent survey highlights the causes in relation to retinopathy changes, which are shown in Table 2.1.

The pattern of blindness in diabetes is that maculopathy is the major cause, particularly in type 2 diabetic subjects, whereas blindness due to proliferative retinopathy is becoming rarer in type 1 diabetes, likely because of the excellent outcomes from laser treatment and modern vitrectomy surgery. It should be noted that the ischaemic form of diabetic maculopathy causes a third of cases of blindness due to maculopathy, and this form is generally untreatable, as laser treatment may be hazardous.

However, blindness in diabetic patients may also due to other conditions, particularly as type 2 diabetes occurs in an older population with other ocular diseases.

In general terms, DR is responsible for approximately 50–60% of blindness in diabetic subjects, whereas the remainder is due to other causes. The major other conditions leading to visual loss are shown in Table 2.1. The pathogenesis of many of these is related to hypertension and lipid disorders, which are associated with diabetes.

While it is of utmost importance to prevent visual loss and blindness in diabetic subjects, the issue is broader than just identifying DR, as there are a number of other different causes. The latter has relevance in screening diabetic populations and identifying these ocular conditions, and in designing protocols needed for their appropriate clinical management (Table 2.2).

Table 2.1 The causes of visual loss due to DR	
Diabetic maculopathy	80%
Non-ischaemic	65%
Ischaemic	35%
Proliferative retinopathy (including vitreous haemorrhage and retinal detachment*)	20%
* Figures are derived before the advent of widespread modern vitrectomy services.	

Table 2.2 **Non-DR causes of visual loss in diabetic subjects**
• Trauma and injury
• Amblyopia
• Age-related macula degeneration
• Retinal vein and artery occlusion, ischaemic optic neuropathy
• Cataract
• Glaucoma
• Hypertension (and macroaneurysms)
• Retinal detachment
• Optic atrophy
• Retinal dystrophies and myopic degeneration.

Table 2.3 **Data showing reduction in severe visual impairment (SVI) due to diabetic retinopathy (DR) over a 12-year period in the diabetic eye clinic in East Birmingham District**

	1992 data N=246	1998 data N=287	2004 data N=471
Duration of the study in months	5	4	5
Number of patients with 8 VI			
All	58 (23.6%)	77 (25.9%)	72 (15.2%)
Diabetic retinopathy	38 (15.5%)	33 (11.1%)	46 (9.7%)
Non-diabetic retinopathy	20 (8.1%)	44 (14.8%)	26 (5.5%)

Data from East Birmingham—M Tahhan et al., 2006. SVI = VA worse than 6/36.

2.3 **Does retinal screening reduce visual loss?**

This is a fundamental question, but, intuitively, screening and treating DR at an early stage when the disease responds best to treatment should provide benefit. The data supporting this comes from three studies. The first showed that by introducing a screening programme along side improved ophthalmic services did indeed reduce the prevalence rate of blindness after 5 years—from 3.5% to 0.5% in type 1 diabetes and 1.1% to 0.6% in type 2 diabetes. There was also a significant reduction of visual loss in both types of diabetes.

The second reported a reduction in rates of blindness and partial sightedness by more than 33% over a 12-year period. Importantly, it took 6 years before a major change in the rates occurred. The third study agrees with these results, demonstrating a reduction of around 33% over a 12-year period (see Table 2.3).

The cost of blindness or partial sightedness is considerable not only in terms of social and welfare costs, but also in terms of financial loss in income during working life (£20 000 per patient registered blind per year). Indeed, visual loss is one of the complications of diabetes most feared by patients.

Both in Europe and the United States, national bodies have assessed the cost-effectiveness of a DR screening programme, and have concluded that screening saves vision for a relatively low cost, and even this cost is often less than the disability payments provided to people who would go blind in the absence of a screening programme (American Diabetes Association statement 1998).

The original St Vincent declaration, reinforced by the more recent Liverpool declaration on DR, supports the value of screening across Europe and has started movement towards this goal.

2.4 **Definition of screening**

The National Screening Committee (NSC) defines screening as a 'public service in which members of a defined population who do not necessarily perceive they are at risk of or are already affected by a disease or its complications, are asked a question or offered a test to identify those individuals who are more likely to be helped than harmed by further tests or treatment to reduce the risk of a disease or its complications'.

The criteria for a successful screening programme are described by Wilson and Jungner (WHO 1968):

- The condition should be an important health problem.
- Its natural history should be well understood.
- There must be a recognized early or latent asymptomatic stage.
- Treatment must be beneficial at an early stage.
- A suitable test must be available.
- This test must be acceptable to the population.
- Adequate facilities must be available for diagnosis and treatment.
- Screening is done at predefined regular intervals.
- The benefits of screening must outweigh the risks, both to the individual and the population as a whole.
- Screening must be cost-effective.

Screening for DR using digital retinal photography fulfils these requirements for a screening programme. DR has important adverse effects; laser treatment is effective, it can be easily detected by digital photography, which is an acceptable test, and is cost-effective.

A national programme spanning the four nations of the United Kingdom is therefore being undertaken and this is equivalent to other national schemes of cervical and breast cancer screening programmes. The details of the DR scheme are described in Chapters 12, 13, and 14.

Appendix

The legal definition of blindness according to the National Assistance Act 1948,

> a person can be registered as blind if they are 'so blind that they cannot do any work for which eyesight is essential'. A person may be registered as partially sighted if they are 'substantially and permanently handicapped by defective vision, caused by congenital defect or illness or injury'.
> (National Assistance Act 1948)

Blindness may be defined as visual acuity (VA) of less than 3/60 or corresponding visual field loss in the better eye with best possible correction. Low vision corresponds to visual acuity of less than 6/18, but equal or better than 3/60 in the better eye with best possible correction (WHO 1990).

Chapter 3

Anatomy of the eye and the healthy fundus

Laurence Quant

Key points

- The anterior segment
  - The cornea
  - The sclera
  - The iris
  - The lens
  - The aqueous humour.
- The posterior segment
  - The vitreous humour
  - The retina
  - The neuro-sensory layer
  - The photoreceptors (rods and cones)
  - The retinal pigment epithelium (RPE)
  - Bruch's membrane
  - The choroid
  - The macula
  - The fovea
  - The retinal vasculature
  - The optic nerve.
- The appearance of a healthy fundus
- Normal variations:
  - Pigmentation
  - RPE changes
  - Glare
  - Pseudophakia
  - Tortuous vessels
  - Tigroid fundus
  - Myopic crescent.

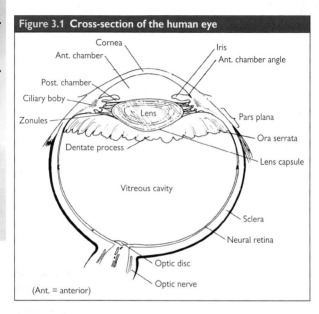

Figure 3.1 Cross-section of the human eye

Cornea
Ant. chamber
Post. chamber
Ciliary boby
Zonules
Dentate process
Iris
Ant. chamber angle
Lens
Pars plana
Ora serrata
Lens capsule
Vitreous cavity
Sclera
Neural retina
Optic disc
Optic nerve

(Ant. = anterior)

3.1 **The anterior segment**

The anterior segment makes up the front third of the eye between the cornea and lens. It includes the cornea, iris, ciliary body, lens, and two spaces filled with aqueous humour: the anterior chamber and the posterior chamber.

The anterior chamber is the space between the innermost surface of the cornea and the anterior surfaces of the iris and lens. The anterior chamber angle is situated peripherally and is home to the trabecular network (comb-like fibres) responsible for most of the outflow of aqueous humour. The posterior chamber is much smaller in comparison. It is the space between the iris posteriorly and the front face of the zonular fibres which suspend the lens in position.

3.1.1 **The cornea**

The cornea is the transparent window at the front of the eye. It is approximately 11.5mm in diameter. Both the cornea and the lens refract light, enabling the eye to focus. The cornea contributes more to the total refraction, but unlike the lens, the curvature of the cornea is fixed and cannot be adjusted to refine the focus. The cornea, along with the sclera, makes up the spherical outer wall of the eyeball. Both are tough and durable, forming a protective barrier against trauma and the invasion of microorganisms into the eye.

3.1.2 **The sclera**

Together with the transparent cornea, the white sclera makes up the tough outer layer of the eye. The thickness of the sclera varies from around 0.3mm to 1mm. Its main functions include protecting against internal and external forces and providing an attachment for the muscles exterior to the globe of the eye. The sclera is strengthened by a haphazard arrangement of collagen fibrils, allowing it to maintain the shape of the globe of the eye.

3.1.3 **The iris**

The iris is the most visible part of the eye. It consists of a pigmented tissue known as stroma. The iris can be strongly pigmented and the colour ranges include browns, hazels, greens, greys, and blues. At the centre of the iris is the pupil, an aperture which can contract using a sphincter muscle running radially through the iris, connected to the stroma, or dilate due to a dilator muscle, also connected to the stroma. The iris has two main functions: controlling light entry to the retina and reducing intra-ocular light scatter.

3.1.4 **The lens**

The lens is a flexible, transparent, biconvex structure composed almost entirely of protein. It is found in the anterior segment of the eye and helps refract light, along with the cornea. Its transparency is achieved because of the fact that it is acellular and also because most of the layers of the lens have the same index of refraction.

By altering the lens curvature, the eye is able to focus on objects at different distances from it. The curvature of the lens is changed and controlled by the circularly arranged ciliary muscle, situated in the uveal part of the ciliary body. Zonular fibres arise from the ciliary body and are inserted into the zonule in the lens, suspending it in position during accommodation. This enables changes in the ciliary muscle to affect lens curvature.

In order to adapt to short range focus, the ciliary muscle contracts, releasing the tension on the lens caused by the zonular fibres, making the lens more convex. In order to increase long range focus the ciliary muscle relaxes, causing the zonular fibres to become taut, flattening the lens.

3.1.5 **The aqueous humour**

The aqueous humour is a thick fluid filling the anterior segment, the space between the cornea and lens. It contributes to the normal maintenance of intra-ocular pressure and helps maintain the convex shape of the cornea. It also contributes to the nutrition of the endothelial layer of the cornea.

The aqueous humour supplies the metabolism of the lens (which is avascular) and carries away the associated waste products. It is secreted by the ciliary processes into the posterior chamber and flows around the margin of the pupil and into the anterior chamber. Around 80% of the aqueous humour drains out from the eye via the trabecular network in the anterior chamber angle, into the Canal of Schlemm. Elsewhere, it is also able to flow via the uveoscleral outflow path, into the potential space between the sclera and ciliary body.

3.2 **The posterior segment**

The posterior segment makes up two-thirds of the eye, from the lens to the back of the eyeball. It includes the vitreous humour, retina, choroid, and optic nerve.

3.2.1 **The vitreous humour**

The vitreous humour is a clear solution with a gel-like consistency found in the area between the lens and retina. It makes up 80% of the globe of the eye and has an average volume of 4mL in an adult eye.

The vitreous humour suspends the lens and provides a cushioned support for the eye, helping to maintain its overall shape. It has a complex structure of collagen fibrils, together with molecules of a high molecular weight. These add to its viscosity and elasticity, preventing rapid flow into and out of the globe, thus maintaining its volume. The visco-elasticity of the vitreous humour also gives it strong water-binding properties (the remaining 99% of the vitreous humour is water) which give it optical clarity by letting light through without introducing further refraction.

The vitreous humour is attached by a circular band straddling the ora serrata and in the area around the margin of the optic disc. The attachment around the optic disc weakens with age, making posterior vitreous attachment more common in the elderly.

3.2.2 **The retina**

The retina is the inner layer of the eye. It covers the inner surface of the eyeball extending from the optic disc to the ora serrata anteriorly. Both the retina and optic nerve start out as outgrowths of the developing brain. The retina is therefore a part of the central nervous system. It consists of two main layers (Figure 3.2), the innermost being the neuro-sensory layer and then the retinal pigment epithelial layer.

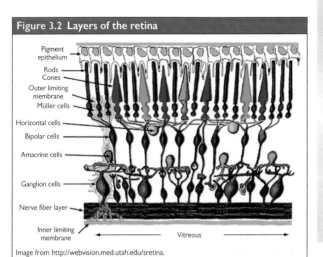

Figure 3.2 Layers of the retina

Pigment epithelium
Rods
Cones
Outer limiting membrane
Müller cells
Horizontal cells
Bipolar cells
Amacrine cells
Ganglion cells
Nerve fiber layer
Inner limiting membrane
Vitreous

Image from http://webvision.med.utah.edu/sretina.

The retina can also be divided into 10 separate, more detailed layers, starting from the layer closest to the vitreous:

1. **The internal limiting membrane** separates the retina from the vitreous. It consists of Müller cells (glial cells), which provide support, protection, nutrition, and oxygen to neurons (the other main type of cell in the nervous system). Müller cells are involved in homeostasis, the forming of myelin and signal transmission. They also remove dead neurons and destroy pathogens.

2. **Axons**: These are long, slender projections of neurons (nerve fibres). They conduct electrical impulses from ganglion cells, across the retina to the optic disc, where they leave the eye.

3. **Ganglion cells**: These are neurons that receive visual information from the photoreceptors.

4. **The inner plexiform layer** consists of axons of bipolar cells and dendrites (branched projections of neurons, conducting electrical stimulation).

5. **The inner nuclear layer** consists of the nuclei of bipolar neurons, horizontal cells, amacrine cells, and Müller cells.

6. **The outer plexiform layer** is composed of axons, rod and cone cells, dendrites of bipolar neurons (horizontal cells and amacrine cells), and Müller cells.

7. **The outer nuclear layer** consists of the nuclei of the rod and cone cells (see photoreceptors).

8. **The external (outer) limiting membrane** comprises junctional complexes between Müller cells and rod and cone cells. It makes up a narrow line slightly internal to the rod and cone outer segments.

9. **The photoreceptor layer** is responsible for receiving light that reaches the retina. The photoreceptor layer is made up of the outer segments of photoreceptor cells (see Section 3.2.4). Cone cells are shorter, darker, and thicker. Rod cells are paler, thinner, and longer.

10. **Retinal pigment epithelium (RPE):** (see Section 3.2.7).

3.2.3 **The neuro-sensory layer**

The neuro-sensory retina is divided into three separate layers. The most internal is a layer of ganglion cells. Next is the inner nuclear layer. This contains intermediate neurons. The most external is the photoreceptor layer. This includes inner and outer segments and a layer of photoreceptor cells.

3.2.4 **Photoreceptor cells**

Photoreceptor cells respond to focused light. There are two kinds of photoreceptor cell: rod and cone cells.

3.2.5 **Rod cells**

The human retina contains about 100 million rod cells. They are around hundred times more sensitive to a single photon of light than cone cells. They are therefore responsible for night vision and function in less intense light. Rod cells are located in the periphery of the retina and diminish in number towards the macula. None are found in the fovea. This makes them also responsible for peripheral vision.

3.2.6 **Cone cells**

The human retina contains about 5 million cone cells. These are mostly concentrated at the macula and fovea (see Sections 3.2.10 and 3.2.11), gradually becoming sparser towards the periphery of the retina. Cone cells function best in bright light and are most responsible for perception of colour, fine visual acuity, and central vision. The response time to visual stimuli is faster with cone cells than with rod cells. This makes cone cells able to perceive finer details and more rapid changes in imagery.

3.2.7 **The retinal pigment epithelium (RPE)**

The RPE is situated between the photoreceptors and their blood supply, known as choriocapillaries. It consists of a single layer of specialist cells known as epithelial cells. The epithelial cells are concerned with the maintenance of the photoreceptors. This involves removal of waste products. The epithelial cells are hexagonal, making the junctions between them a tight blood barrier.

3.2.8 **Bruch's membrane**

Bruch's membrane provides support for the retina. It consists of five layers:

1. Basement membrane of the RPE
2. Inner collagenous zone
3. Central band of elastic fibres
4. Outer collagenous zone
5. Basement membrane of the choriocapillaries.

As the RPE transports metabolic waste from the photoreceptors, these cross Bruch's membrane into the choroid. Thickening of Bruch's membrane with age slows the transportation of these metabolites which may, in turn, lead to the formation of drusen (see Chapter 9) and age-related macular degeneration.

3.2.9 **The choroid**

The choroid is a vascular layer, lying between the retina and sclera. Smaller capillary blood vessels (choriocapillaries) form a dense network adjacent to the retina, whilst the vessels situated closer to the sclera are larger. The choroid provides oxygen and nourishment to the outer retinal layers whilst removing the metabolites generated by the retinal photoreceptors. The choroid helps limit reflections within the eye that would otherwise confuse the perception of images. The red-reflex in retinal photography and red-eye effect in portrait photography are caused by reflection of light from the choroid.

3.2.10 **The macula**

The macula is the area of the retina within 2-disc diameter (2DD) of the centre of the fovea (see Chapter 6 for definitions). It is a precious region, carefully observed during retinopathy screening because of the high proportion of cone cells: photoreceptors responsible for visual acuity, colour, and central vision. It is highly specialized, and light falling on the macula occupies a substantial portion of the brain's visual capacity.

3.2.11 **The fovea**

Across the retina, light must pass through all the intervening layers to reach the outer segments of the photoreceptor cells. This is not the case at the fovea, which, as the central part of the macula has a high proportion of cone cells.

3.2.12 **The retinal vasculature**

The retinal vasculature enters and leaves the eye through the optic disc in the form of the central retinal artery and vein. These branch into four main arterial and venous trunks or 'arcades', which run in the nerve fibre layer and supply each quadrant of the retina. Retinal circulation is controlled by auto-regulation, which maintains a constant blood flow, and is triggered by acute changes in oxygen and major changes in perfusion pressure.

3.2.13 **The optic nerve**

The optic nerve connects the eye to the brain and is considered part of the central nervous system, covered with a myelin sheath. It is composed of retinal ganglion cell axons and support cells. The optic nerve contains around 1.2 million nerve fibres which run from the retina to nine primary visual nuclei in the brain. Visual information is transmitted along these fibres.

The head of the optic nerve is called the optic disc. It is about 1.5mm in diameter. The optic disc comprises a whitish-yellow, funnel-shaped depression called the central cup and a surrounding neural rim. A healthy neural rim is pinkish orange because of a rich network of capillaries and has a clearly defined margin. The eye has a blind spot resulting from the absence of retina at the optic disc.

3.3 **The appearance of a healthy fundus**

The retina forms the inner layer of the eye. Retinal appearances differ and colouration varies from intense oranges to deeper reddish browns. It is normal for a fundus to appear lighter and brighter in some places and duller in others. In terms of layout, the right and left eyes are usually mirror images of one another, with the optic disc positioned on the nasal side in both eyes.

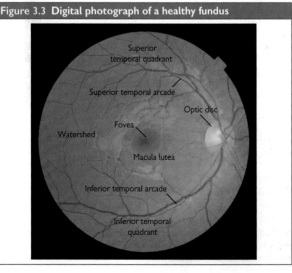

Figure 3.3 **Digital photograph of a healthy fundus**

Macula-centred view: When looking at a fundus photograph, the side closest to the nose is referred to as nasal and the side furthest away is known as temporal. These terms can either be used to describe regions or 'quadrants' of the fundus, or to describe navigation around the fundus.

The examples in Figure 3.3 and 3.4 are identifiable as a right eye because the optic disc, which is always on the nasal side, is to the right of the fovea. If the photograph were of a left eye, the layout would be close to a mirror image in layout. This means nasal and temporal would be on the opposite sides and the optic disc would be to the left of the fovea.

Figure 3.4 Nasal view of the same fundus, with the optic disc in the centre

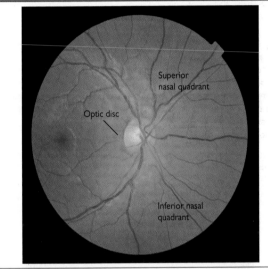

Superior nasal quadrant

Optic disc

Inferior nasal quadrant

The optic disc is the head of the optic nerve and the most obvious landmark on the fundus. It is yellow in appearance and about 1.5mm in diameter. Visible features include a whitish-yellow, funnel-shaped depression called the central cup and a surrounding neural rim. A healthy neural rim is pinkish-orange and has a clearly defined margin.

The optic disc forms a central point for the retinal blood vessels. A superior and inferior arcade, each with arterioles and veins, can be seen arching around the fundus, temporal to the optic disc. The pattern and branching of the inferior arcade roughly mirrors that of the superior arcade. The nasal vessels are similarly mirrored; however, they simply radiate from the optic disc, as opposed to arching. Finer, single vessels can also be seen at the disc. In a healthy fundus, these follow a logical path, without excessive deviation.

Retinal veins appear a deeper red than arteries because of the relative lack of oxygenation of the blood. The exact shape, calibre, and relationship of the veins and arterioles in each arcade varies. The calibre ratio of veins in relation to arteries should be around 3:2. In digital photography, a white streak of glare is often seen running along vessels. It is caused by reflection from the flash and is more distinct on arteries than on veins. If sporadic, it can be mistaken for cholesterol emboli.

Temporal to the optic disc is the macula, an area appearing darker than the surrounding retina. The central point of the macula is the fovea, an important area for central and colour vision. The fovea appears yellow due to luteal pigment.

3.4 **Normal variations**

3.4.1 **Pigmentation**
Retinal colouring depends on ethnicity.

Figure 3.5 Pigmentation: white, caucasion fundus (left eye, macula centred). A caucasian retina usually has a range of red, orange, and pink tones

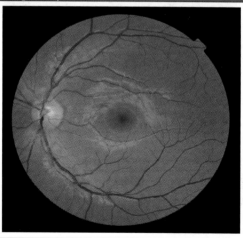

3.4.2 Tigroid fundus

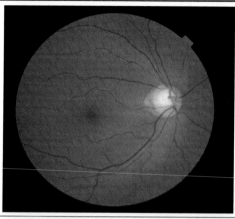

Figure 3.6 A South-Asian fundus (right eye, macula-centred). South-Asian and Afro-Caribbean retinas usually also include darker reds and golden browns

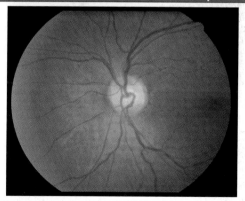

Figure 3.7 Tigroid fundus (left eye, nasal view)—the light stripes result from the choroid visible from beneath the retina, and is common in Afro-Caribbean subjects

The choroidal vessels may be visible from beneath the retina. Sometimes a fundus appears stripy or 'tigroid', with a strong contrast between light and dark. This is because the retina is thin and blood vessels in the choroidal layer can be seen more clearly.

3.4.3 **Myelinated nerve fibres**

Myelin consists of lipid and protein and sheaths of nerve fibres. Its function is to increase the speed of impulses that travel along the nerve fibre. Areas of myelinated nerve fibres can often be seen running along the temporal arcades, creating pale, whitish-yellow streaks. The colouring showing through between them can appear blotchy, as if microaneurysms are present.

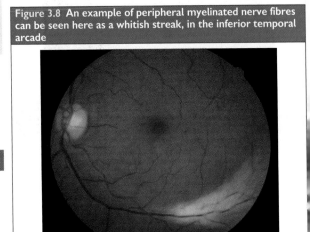

Figure 3.8 An example of peripheral myelinated nerve fibres can be seen here as a whitish streak, in the inferior temporal arcade

3.4.4 **Retinal pigment epithelial (RPE) changes**

Dark or pale pigmentary changes may be visible in the RPE (see Figure 3.9). This is the layer of the retina involved in photoreceptor renewal and removal of the related waste products.

Figure 3.9 RPE changes

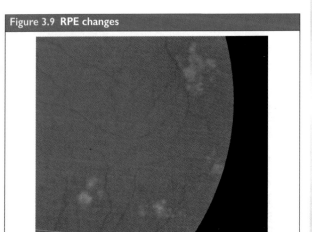

Figure 3.10 Pigment spot—dark brown pigment spots are common. They may be mistaken for microaneurysms or haemorrhages (see Chapter 5), but are not as red in colour

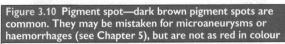

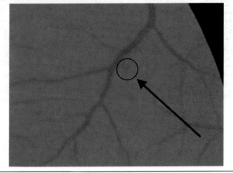

3.4.5 **Reflection and glare**

In digital fundus photography, areas of glare or reflection artefact are common around the macula and temporal arcades (see Figure 3.11). Glare is pale or translucent and can range from white-grey to yellow in colour. It can form wispy patterns or cover whole areas. The reflection results from the incoming light from the flash required for photography. A degree of glare is usual with younger individuals as they have more reflective fundi.

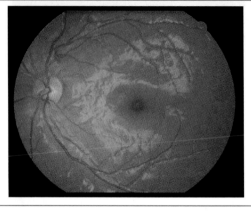

Figure 3.11 Glare—light patches caused by reflection of camera flash

Glare can mask or be confused with pathology—meaning extra caution is required. Comparing macula-centred and nasal views can help a screener/grader decide whether it is glare artefact resulting from the photography process or real pathology—if the pale area changes or has disappeared on the other view then it is generally artefactual and therefore not significant retinopathy.

Widespread glare covering the macula region generally stops to form a circle around the fovea, where small blotches of glare forming foveal reflex are common. Again, these will usually differ between the macula-centred and nasal views.

3.4.6 **Pseudophakia**

If a patient has had cataracts removed and intra-ocular lenses fitted (pseudophakia), their retina appears a paler, more washed out pink. In pseudophakia, small patches of glare can be present, mostly in or around the macula region (see Figure 3.12). These are generally very pale and insubstantial. Their pattern is fairly random and often more subtle.

3.4.7 **Tortuous vessels**

Retinal vessels can appear tortuous (convoluted or willowy) in an individual with hypertension or an impending occlusion; however, if the vein calibre is normal and the retina appears otherwise healthy, this can be a normal variation (see Figure 3.13). Vessels can also become tortuous in pregnancy, returning to normal after delivery.

Figure 3.12 Areas of glare commonly seen with pseudophakia

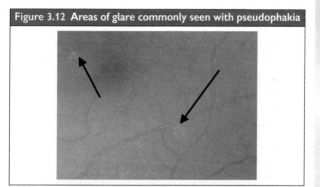

Figure 3.13 Tortuous vessels

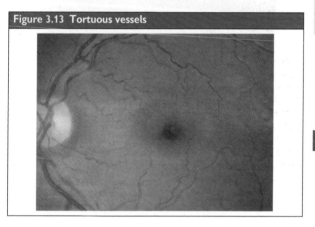

3.4.8 **Myopic crescent and macula changes**

If an individual is short-sighted (myopic), a pale, well-defined myopic crescent can be present around the disc (see Figure 3.14). This is an atrophic area (wasted away) and choroidal vessels clearly show through from beneath the retina. Myopic crescents vary in size, depending on the extent of myopia. Myopic degeneration may also occur in the retina and macula regions.

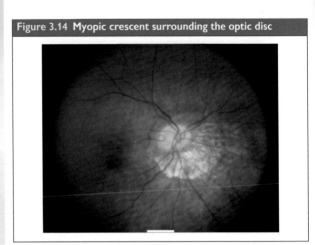

Figure 3.14 Myopic crescent surrounding the optic disc

The retinal features described in this section reflect the diversity of the normal appearance of a retina which must be recognized by all those involved in the screening process. Experience and pattern recognition are key to identifying these retinal changes.

Chapter 4

Diabetes and the eye

Paul M Dodson

Key points

- Diabetes mellitus is still one of the commonest causes of blindness worldwide.
- The ophthalmic complications of diabetes include diabetic retinopathy, cataracts, primary open angle and neovascular glaucoma, and cranial nerve palsies.
- Retinovascular disease including retinal vein and artery occlusion and non-arteritic ischaemic optic neuropathy are more common in diabetic subjects.
- Diabetic retinopathy occurs in approximately 40% of diabetic subjects, with ethnic differences.
- The primary abnormalities of diabetic retinopathy are capillary basement membrane thickening, such that it becomes porous, and capillary occlusion with resultant retinal ischaemia.
- In type 1 diabetes diabetic retinopathy is almost invariable after 15 years of disease duration. In type 2 diabetes 20% have retinal signs at diagnosis of diabetes, rising to a prevalence of 60% after 15 years of known disease duration.
- Major modifiable risk factors for diabetic retinopathy include poor glucose and blood pressure control and increasing lipid levels.

4.1 Ocular complications of diabetes

Whilst diabetic retinopathy (DR) is the most recognized ocular complication, the non-DR changes may cause up to 50% of cases of blindness in diabetic subjects. Table 4.1 shows the major conditions that occur in clinical practice.

Table 4.1 Ocular effects of diabetes

Visual change due to
- Hyperglycaemia leading to refractive changes
- Cataract
- DR:
  - Background
  - Maculopathy
    —*Exudative*
    —*Ischaemic*
    —*Mixed exudative and ischaemic*
    —*Cystoid*
  - Pre-proliferative
  - Proliferative
- Glaucoma
  - Primary open angle and rubeotic
- Cranial nerve palsies (third and sixth nerve) leading to diplopia
- Retinovascular disease
  - Retinal vein and artery occlusion
  - Ischaemic optic neuropathy
- Diabetic papillopathy

Type 2 diabetes may present with blurring of vision due to increased myopia (short sight), resulting from overhydration and swelling of the lens secondary to prolonged hyperglycaemia. These refractive changes reverse as the blood glucose normalizes. It is prudent, however, to delay prescription of glasses for these patients by about 3 months to ensure the metabolic effects are fully resolved.

4.2 **Cataract**

The most common ocular effect of diabetes is of the lens, with resultant cataract formation. This leads to earlier lens opacity formation and more rapid progression. Cataract affects 60% of older onset diabetic patients (aged 30–54 years) compared to 12% of non-diabetic controls. There are three likely pathogenetic mechanisms. The polyol pathway results in increased glucose conversion by aldose reductase to sorbitol which sets up an osmotic gradient. This results in movement of water into the cells of the lens which swell and rupture with opacity formation. Hyperglycaemia also results in increased glycation of lens proteins and excess free radical formation leading to irreversible lens cell damage.

Figure 4.1 Types of cataract

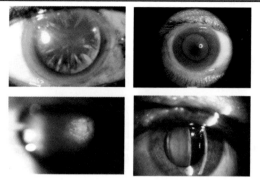

Top left, cortical cataract; top right, white complete lens opacity.
Bottom left, posterior subcapsular lens opacity; bottom right, nuclear lens opacity.

Cortical cataract formation is the most frequent with typical radial spoke-like opacities. Nuclear and subcapsular (anterior or posterior) cataracts may result in reduction and blurring of vision, as well as problems with headlights of oncoming cars and bright sunlight. True diabetic cataract is a result of osmotic overhydration of the lens and appears as bilateral white snowflake opacities and these may mature over days.

4.3 Retinovascular disease

Retinovascular disease is more common in diabetic subjects, largely because of the excess of cardiovascular risk factors which are involved in the aetiology in diabetics. Examples are shown in Figure 4.2.

The aetiology of retinal vein occlusion (RVO) is multifactorial, but the primary event is damage to the wall of the venous vasculature. The major risk factors are hypertension and hyperlipidaemia, which are strongly associated with diabetes.

Figure 4.2 Left panel shows a central retinal vein occlusion and the right panel, the branch form

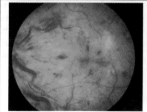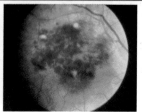

Retinal artery occlusion occurs in both the central and branch form but is less common than RVO and relates to the same risk factors as RVO but is also strongly related to cigarette smoking. Examples of retinal artery occlusion are shown in Figure 4.3.

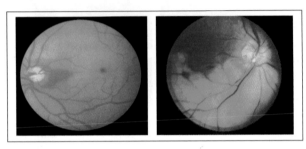

Figure 4.3 Left panel shows an acute central retinal artery occlusion and the right panel a branch retinal artery occlusion due to a cholesterol embolus blocking the inferior temporal artery.

Non-arteritic ischaemic optic neuropathy occurs when there is occlusion to the posterior ciliary artery supply to the optic nerve, resulting in painless visual loss in the form of an altitudinal field defect. A typical retinal appearance is shown in Figure 4.4. The risk factors are similar to retinal artery occlusion.

Figure 4.4 Ischaemic optic neuropathy with swelling of the optic nerve head

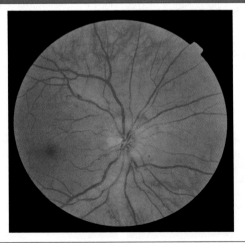

Retinovascular disease is an important cause of visual loss in diabetic subjects. Tight control of cardiovascular risk factors is important to help in prevention as well as avoiding recurrence in the fellow eye with potential disastrous visual outcome.

4.4 **Glaucoma**

Primary open-angle glaucoma (POAG) is increased in the diabetic population. This may lead to visual loss due to progressive loss of optic nerve fibres. This is because of direct injury due to raised intra-ocular pressure, or progressive infarction of the microcirculation of the optic nerve head. The typical sign of classical glaucoma is cupping of the optic disc (see Figure 4.5).

Glaucoma may also be due to advanced diabetic eye disease with growth of new vessels on the iris, termed iris neovascularization (iris rubeosis). The neovascularization of the iris obstructs the drainage angle of the eye (the Canal of Schlemm) and is accompanied by fibrosis leading to rubeotic glaucoma and particularly high intra-ocular pressure. The optic nerve rapidly atrophies and the eye may become rapidly painful.

Figure 4.5 Cupping of the optic disc (left panel) and new vessels on the surface of the iris, termed iris rubeosis or iris neovascularization (right panel)

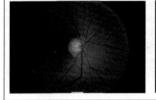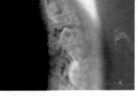

4.5 **Cranial nerve palsies**

Neuropathy of the III, IV, and VI cranial nerves may result in extra-ocular muscle palsies which may be the presentation of undiagnosed diabetes mellitus. These present with double vision (diplopia), usually painless, and will slowly resolve within 6 months of onset. The pathology is segmental demyelination of the affected nerve secondary to ischaemia produced by microangiopathy (small-vessel disease).

4.6 **Diabetic retinopathy**

Diabetic small-vessel disease (diabetic microangiopathy) is a specific, but at the same time generalized, disorder of small blood vessels. It is specific in that it only occurs in patients with diabetes, but generalized in that it can appear in virtually every small vessel in the body. The histological hallmark of microangiopathy is capillary basement membrane thickening. In addition, the basement membrane architecture becomes abnormal and porous, causing leakage of plasma protein that in turn leads to the development of profound abnormalities within the microcirculation. The principal vascular beds that are affected include the eyes (retinopathy), the kidneys (nephropathy), and the neurovascular bundle of peripheral nerves (neuropathy).

Hyperglycaemia affects retinal blood flow and metabolism and has a direct effect on the cells associated with the retinal circulation. There is loss of retinal pericytes in the capillary walls, which are needed to maintain retinal vascular autoregulation of blood flow, and the endothelial cell lining.

Although the pathogenetic role of hyperglycaemia is proven, it is not known precisely how glucose toxicity results in retinopathy; but there are a number of potential effects on the retinal perfusion which result in vascular leakage and retinal ischaemia and summarized in Figure 4.6. A stained histological preparation of a retina with diabetic changes is shown in Figure 4.7 demonstrating the formation of microaneurysms and capillary closure. An exact description of the stages of DR is given in detail in later chapters.

The consequences of hyperglycaemia include capillary cell death, alteration of retinal pericyte/endothelial cell ratio, and vascular occlusion. Increased blood flow in the capillaries occurs because of loss of pericytes in the normal retina, leading to disruption of retinal blood flow autoregulation. The resulting increased blood flow affects the capillary wall by stimulating production of vaso-active substances and increasing endothelial cell proliferation, eventually resulting in the closure of the capillary circulation. This leads to a state of chronic hypoxia (low oxygen) in the retina and increase in the levels of a number of growth factors, including vascular endothelial growth factor (VEGF), insulin-like growth factor 1 (IGF-1), and fibroblast growth factor (FGF) (see also Chapter 7, section 7.3.1).

Figure 4.6 An illustration of the changes that occur in the development of diabetic retinopathy (DR) and pathogenetic factors

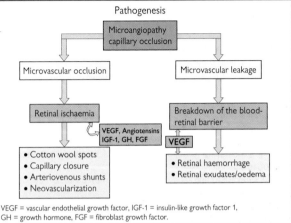

Pathogenesis

Microangiopathy capillary occlusion

Microvascular occlusion → Retinal ischaemia

VEGF, Angiotensins IGF-1, GH, FGF

- Cotton wool spots
- Capillary closure
- Arteriovenous shunts
- Neovascularization

Microvascular leakage → Breakdown of the blood-retinal barrier

VEGF

- Retinal haemorrhage
- Retinal exudates/oedema

VEGF = vascular endothelial growth factor, IGF-1 = insulin-like growth factor 1, GH = growth hormone, FGF = fibroblast growth factor.

Figure 4.7 A stain of a retinal section outlining the vasculature and key changes in DR

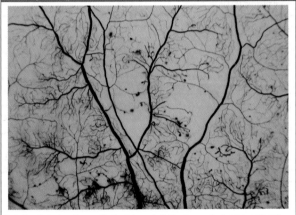

Retinal capillaries have been outlined and demonstrate the changes of microaneurysms and areas of capillary non-perfusion.

4.7 **Epidemiology and risk factors for DR**

DR is one of the most common causes of blindness in the working population of the developed world and a significant cause of blindness in the elderly population. The risk of DR increases with disease duration. Epidemiological studies have shown that the prevalence of DR is greater than 95% after 15 years of disease in patients diagnosed with diabetes before the age of 30 (principally type 1 diabetes). Of those diagnosed after that age (principally type 2 diabetes), 20% have signs of retinopathy at diagnosis. In the United Kingdom, around 40% of all patients with diabetes have DR, 2% are partially sighted or blind, and approximately 400 new cases of blindness are registered every year.

Recent data from the digital camera DR Screening Programme has demonstrated more accurate prevalence rates with approximately 40% of all diabetics having some form of DR and 5% with sight-threatening maculopathy.

Ethnic differences are apparent with an increased rate of retinopathy and maculopathy in diabetic patients of Asian or Afro-Carribbean origin, as shown in Figure 4.8.

	Established (A)	New digital (B)	Asian (C)
Normal (R0)	57%	47%	54.4%
Maculopathy (M1)	5%	7.5%	12.7%
Preproliferative (R2)	3%	1.1%	1%
Proliferative (R3)	1%	1.2%	3%
Referral rate	7.8%	10%	16.4%
Ungradable	1.8%	2%	—

The R system (R0, R1, R2, R3) are the retinopathy levels used in the English Diabetic Retinopathy Screening Programme (see Chapter 11).

Figure 4.8 Prevalence rates of DR and referral rates for a well-established digital camera screened diabetic population (A), a newly digitally screened population (B) in South Birmingham, and from the UK Asian study (C) in Birmingham and Coventry.

There are differences between the two types of diabetes. In type 1 diabetes, DR is almost invariable with greater than 95% affected after 15 years duration. In contrast, 20% have signs of DR at diagnosis of type 2 diabetes, rising to 60% after 15 years known diagnosis (see Figure 4.9).

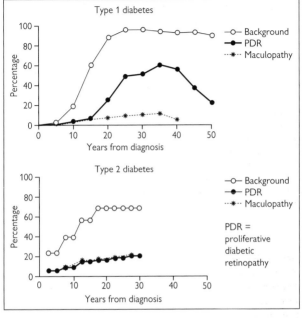

Figure 4.9 The prevalence of DR in type 1 and type 2 diabetes demonstrating the tight relationship with increasing duration in both types

In children with type 1 diabetes, it is unusual to observe DR before 8 years of diabetes duration, such that the youngest diabetic patient reported with retinopathy in the literature is after 11 years of age. Whilst there is an increased prevalence related to puberty, the recommended age to start screening for DR has therefore been set to >12 years. However, diabetes now presents in babies and, therefore, individual decisions will need to be made as to when to start DR screening.

With regard to type of DR, 50% of patients with type 1 diabetes, and approximately 10% of those with type 2 diabetes may develop proliferative DR after 15 years known duration of the disease. Whilst around 5% of patients in cross-sectional studies will need to be referred for ophthalmological examination because of sight-threatening maculopathy,

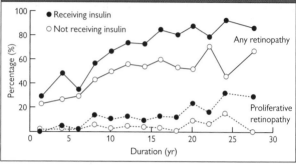

Figure 4.10 The prevalence of DR (%) in those on insulin compared to those not on insulin and the relationship to duration of diabetes

the incidence of macular oedema over a period of 10 years is 20% in type 1 diabetic subjects, and 25% in type 2 patients requiring insulin versus 13.9% in type 2 diabetic patients who did not. The latter reinforces the importance of insulin therapy as shown in Figure 4.10. This also demonstrates the crucial role of increasing duration of diabetes in the development of DR.

Note that in general

- Proliferative retinopathy is more common in type 1 diabetes.
- Maculopathy is more strongly associated with type 2 diabetes.
- 80% of cases registered visually impaired or blind because of DR are due to diabetic maculopathy.
- Modern management of type 1 diabetes and appropriate ophthalmological care, including timely vitrectomy surgery, have resulted in blindness due to proliferative retinopathy being relatively rare.

4.7.1 Risk factors for development of DR

The risk factors for development of DR are

- Increasing duration of diabetes mellitus
- Type of diabetes (more common in type 1 diabetes than type 2)
- Increased blood pressure
- Poor glycaemic control
- Presence of macro- or microalbuminuria
- Increasing serum cholesterol levels
- Pregnancy
- Cigarette smoking.

The first two risk factors listed, increased duration and type of diabetes are non-modifiable but the others listed are modifiable, such that medical management is aimed at optimizing glycaemic and blood pressure control, with attention to lipid levels and cessation of cigarette smoking as outlined in Chapters 1 and 16.

Epidemiological studies have also confirmed that increasing serum cholesterol and triglyceride levels are related to the development of macular exudation, macular oedema, and proliferative retinopathy; see Figure 4.11.

The presence of micro- or macroalbuminuria is a strong predictor of DR, not surprising in that it too is a microvascular complication with similar risk factors, and is also common in both type 1 and 2 diabetics.

Diabetic pregnancy is a definite risk factor for increased progression of DR, as reports have shown that DR may progress with visual loss during pregnancy. The predictive factors for deterioration include the presence of proteinuria and pre-existing retinopathy changes before pregnancy.

The relationship between smoking and retinopathy is unclear as some studies have shown smoking to be an adverse factor, whilst others have almost suggested cigarette smoking to be protective.

Whilst genetic influences may have a role in diabetic nephropathy, there is some weak evidence to suggest that there could be a genetic component. Familial clustering of severe vision-threatening DR was

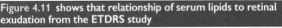

Figure 4.11 shows that relationship of serum lipids to retinal exudation from the ETDRS study

43

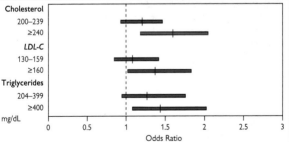

Cholesterol
200–239
≥240
LDL-C
130–159
≥160
Triglycerides
204–399
≥400
mg/dL

0   0.5   1   1.5   2   2.5   3
Odds Ratio

Note: Controlling for other independent risk factors in multiple logistic regression models. ETDRS = Early Treatment Diabetic Retinopathy Study. LDL-C = low density Lipoprotein cholesterol.

observed in the DCCT trial and the continued progression of DR after institution of normoglycaemia may be consistent with altered critical gene expression induced by chronic hyperglycaemia.

Special circumstances are relevant to clinical care. It is well established that DR may deteriorate with a rapid and major improvement in glycaemic control. This is common following the institution of insulin therapy, therefore leading to the requirement for more frequent retinal examination. Although the mechanism of the deterioration is not clear, there is benefit of improved glycaemic control in the longer term. Patients with diabetic nephropathy also have a higher risk of deterioration, such that patients either approaching dialysis or with a low glomerular filtration rate (GFR) should be more frequently monitored.

Further reading

Beri MR, Klugman MR, Kohler JA, Mayren SS (1987). Anterior ischaemic optic neuropathy; incidence of bilaterality and various influencing factors. *Ophthalmology*, **94**: 1020–8.

Broadbent DM, Scott JA, Vora JP, *et al.* (1999). Prevalence of diabetic eye disease in an inner city population: the Liverpool Diabetic Eye Study. *Eye*, **13**: 160–5.

Chowdhury TA, Hopkins D, Dodson PM, *et al.* (2002). The role of serum lipids in exudative diabetic maculopathy: is there a place for lipid lowering therapy? *Eye,* **16**: 689–93.

Dodson PM, Gibson JM, Kritzinger EE (1995). Clinical retinopathies, Chapter 7—retinal artery occlusion & Chapter 8—retinal vein occlusion. Chapman and Hall, London.

Donaldson M and Dodson PM, (2003). Medical treatment of diabetic retinopathy. *Eye*, **17**: 550–62.

Frank RN (2004). Diabetic retinopathy. *New England Journal of Medicine*, 350: 48–58.

Klein R, Klein BE, Moss SE, *et al.* (1998). The Wisconsin Epidemiologic Study of Diabetic Retinopathy: XVII. The 14-year incidence and progression of diabetic retinopathy and associated risk factors in type 1 diabetes. *Ophthalmology*, **105**: 1801–15.

Klein R, Klein BE, Moss SE, *et al.* (1984). The Wisconsin Epidemiologic Study of Diabetic Retinopathy 111. The prevalence and risk of diabetic retinopathy when age at diagnosis is 30 years or more years. *Archives of Ophthalmology*, **102**: 527–32.

Klein B, Moss SE, Klein R (1990). The effect of pregnancy on the progression of diabetic retinopathy. *Diabetes Care*,**13**: 34.

Prasad S, Kamath GG, Jones K, *et al.* (2001). Prevalence of blindness and visual impairment in a population of people with diabetes. *Eye*, **15**: 640–3.

Chapter 5

Background diabetic retinopathy

Laurence Quant

Key points

- Background diabetic retinopathy consists of
  - Microaneurysms
  - Haemorrhages
  - Exudation
  - Cotton wool spots
- Background changes are, as its name suggests, not visually threatening
- Background changes if identified for the first time, are a warning sign that microvascular disease is present.
- Back ground changes are common, affecting up to 40% of the diabetic population.

5.1 Background diabetic retinopathy

Background diabetic retinopathy is the term used for diabetic retinopathy (DR) in its earliest and least sight-threatening forms. It is either less developed than other referable stages of retinopathy or found further away from the fovea and therefore marks less of a threat to central vision.

Background diabetic retinopathy does not in itself disrupt visual function. Presence of any of the main features—microaneurysms, haemorrhages, exudate, or cotton wool spots—does indicate, however, a susceptibility to further retinal damage. A referral to ophthalmology is not necessary at this stage but attention to blood glucose and blood pressure control is important.

5.2 Microaneurysms

Microaneurysms (see Figure 5.1) are commonly found in the early stages of diabetic retinopathy. Weakening of the capillary wall forms small red dots which become visible in the retina. These may be single or more

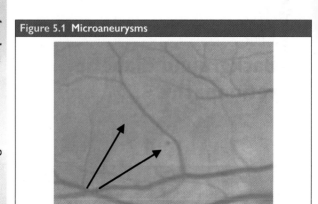

Figure 5.1 Microaneurysms

widespread across the fundus. Microaneurysms are usually clearly identifiable; however, they can be similar in appearance to end on vessels (vessels rising up through the retinal vasculature, rather than along the retina) or colour variations of a healthy fundus. They are usually discrete from the main vessels and are distinct in appearance.

On their own, microaneurysms constitute little threat to vision. If, however, there is a deterioration in visual acuity (VA) to 6/12 or worse, and microaneurysms are present in the macula, then this ceases to be background retinopathy and a referral to ophthalmology is needed (see Chapter 6).

5.3 **Haemorrhages**

Haemorrhages are commonly seen in DR, although some have other causes such as valsalva (rise in pressure of the chest cavity due to straining such as in coughing or constipation) or systemic conditions (e.g. anaemia, leukaemia). In background diabetic retinopathy, intra-retinal haemorrhages originate from ruptured capillaries within the retina. These capillaries are deeper than microaneurysms and the circumference of haemorrhage is usually greater as a result. Intra-retinal haemorrhages are roughly round in appearance and are often described as 'dot' or 'blot' haemorrhages. As with the other main forms of background diabetic retinopathy, the haemorrhages themselves do not disturb visual function. Both haemorrhages and microaneurysms can increase or resolve over time.

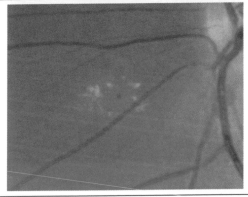

Figure 5.2 A ring of exudate leaking from a solitary microaneurysm

5.4 Exudation

Exudation is a lipoprotein residue found in the retina as a result of oedema. It leaks into the retina as a result of changes in the retinal vessels. Exudate (see Figure 5.2) is yellow and waxy and, in digital fundus photography, appears to be on top of the retina, as opposed to within it. This, combined with its well-defined edges, helps differentiation from retinal pigment epithelium (RPE) change or reflection. Exudate may appear in a variety of patterns, including individual patches, tracking lines, circinates, and macular stars. Many of these formations occur more commonly in the macula region constituting maculopathy, (see Chapter 6). Outside the macula, exudates are most commonly seen in small patches, clumps, and circinates.

47

5.5 Cotton wool spots

Cotton wool spots are ischaemic (caused by a lack of blood) lesions due to disruption of normal axoplasmic flow within the nerve fibre layer of the retina (see Figure 5.3). They are caused by a localized failure of the capillary network to supply oxygen. Cotton wool spots have a characteristic fluffy, white appearance (hence their name), which fades over time. In digital photography, this fluffy appearance generally makes them clearly identifiable, although they may resemble RPE change or reflection.

Figure 5.3 Cotton wool spot

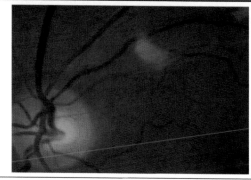

Cotton wool spots may occur on their own or with other features of DR such as microaneurysms and haemorrhages. Data from studies have suggested that up to five cotton wool spots in a retina constitute background diabetic retinopathy. Care needs to be taken when screening, as they are often present in pre-proliferative DR (see Chapter 7, Figures 7.1 and 7.2). A number of other conditions also cause cotton wool spots, notably hypertension, pregnancy, and the contraceptive pill.

Background diabetic retinopathy is not in itself sight threatening. It is an indicator of early microvascular disease, but is at a stage when annual recall for screening is still the outcome of the screening event (the same outcome as if no retinopathy is present). Many of the same features, such as microaneurysms and cotton wool spots, can constitute referable retinopathy in different circumstances (see Chapters 6 and 7) and retinal screeners should have a clear grasp of why the pathology discovered is classified as background and what can change a grade from background retinopathy to maculopathy or pre-proliferative DR.

Further reading

Butcher A and Dodson PM (2001). Chapter 9 pages 119–131. In Sinclair AJ and Finucane P, eds. *Diabetes in old age*. John Wiley & Sons Ltd, Chicester.

Dodson PM, Gibson JM, Kritzinger EE (1995). Chapter 4 pages 38–39. In *Clinical retinopathies*. Chapman and Hall, London.

Chapter 6

Maculopathy

Rebecca Lone

Key points

- Maculopathy is one of the commonest causes of blindness in the Western world.
- In diabetic populations diabetic maculopathy causes blindness in 80% of cases due to diabetic retinopathy (DR).
- It is defined as a disease of the macula region located within the retina.
- Screening for diabetic maculopathy and identification of surrogate markers for clinically significant macula oedema (CSMO) will identify sight-threatening maculopathy at a stage when there is the best potential laser treatment outcome.
- There are three main types of maculopathy: exudative, ischaemic, and cystoid maculopathy due to diabetes, all of which have a detrimental effect on visual acuity (VA) if untreated.

6.1 Introduction to diabetic maculopathy

Diabetic maculopathy is the commonest cause of blindness due to retinopathy from diabetes. It accounts for a large percentage particularly in type 2 diabetic patients. A cross-sectional study identified that the prevalence of diabetic maculopathy was 15% for type 1 patients and 23% for type 2 patients. Furthermore, of those patients who had background retinopathy the prevalence of maculopathy was remarkably high, 42% in type 1 patients and 53% in type 2 patients. Maculopathy carries a very high risk of loss in central vision; its direct relationship is shown in various studies, indicating a decrease in visual acuity (VA) with increasing severity of diabetic maculopathy. This emphasizes the importance of screening for diabetic maculopathy as it is an asymptomatic disease in the earlier stages of development. This is exactly the stage that has the best visual outcome resulting from laser treatment.

6.1.1 **Anatomical features of the macula**

The macula region of the retina is defined as a circular area of 2 disc diameters (2DD) centred on the fovea (Figure 6.1). The fovea is located 2.5DD temporal to the optic disc. The macula appears as a darker circular area due to different pigmentation compared to the peripheral retina. It is highly sensitive and is primarily responsible for central vision. Within the centre of the macula lies a pit known as the fovea. The fovea is the thinnest part of the retina and consists of a high concentration of cone cells which are responsible for central vision, fine VA, and colour vision (see Chapter 3). Diabetic changes such as microaneurysms, exudates, or oedema in this area will most likely affect vision due to disruption of the arrangement of photoreceptors. This can affect central VA, resulting in blurring of vision, and can be recorded on VA testing.

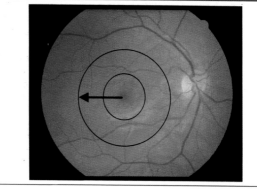

Figure 6.1 Anatomical area of the macula. The inner circle indicates 1DD from the fovea and the outer circle indicates 2DD from the fovea (macula region)

6.1.2 **Development of diabetic maculopathy**

Diabetic maculopathy is a disease of the macula which occurs because diabetes alters the physical properties of the retinal vasculature. Changes in blood flow due to hyperglycaemia lead to vascular changes within the small vessels, resulting in vascular abnormalities that disrupt vascular flow. As the basement membrane thickens, this causes the loss of pericytes from retinal vessel walls. Pericytes are contractile cells that control vascular blood flow via autoregulation. The loss of control increases the blood flow and pressure within the vessel lumen, leading to the loss of tight junctions in the endothelial wall which maintain the blood-retinal barrier, hence increasing blood flow and capillary permeability. Changes in the vascular structure of the vessel endothelium and blood flow lead to the capillary leakage of blood, lipids, protein, and water. The breakdown of the endothelial wall leads to the early clinical signs seen in diabetic maculopathy such as exudates and macula oedema (exudative maculopathy). Capillary closure will also occur at an advanced stage because of increased perfusion pressure at the capillaries causing infiltration of cells and swelling which causes blockage and resultant macula ischaemia (ischaemic maculopathy).

6.1.3 Screening for diabetic maculopathy

Detection of diabetic changes in the macula using two-dimensional (2D) digital images allows identification of sight-threatening retinopathy. Macula oedema and retinal thickening will not be detected on 2D views but require a three-dimensional (3D) view as is performed on slit lamp biomicroscopy examination. Therefore, macula oedema is difficult to distinguish on a 2D flat digital image. It is, therefore, necessary to identify macula changes present on a 2D view that strongly correlates and predicts the presence of macula oedema. Following a literature review, a grading committee advised the following retinal changes to be the best surrogate markers (approximately 10% will have macula oedema), and this has been incorporated into the National Screening Committee (NSC) recommendations.

Central vision may be affected once macula oedema develops, by disrupting the regular arrangement of the photoreceptors. However, it should be noted that there is only a limited correlation between the degree of macula oedema and visual loss. In summary, the surrogate markers stipulated by the NSC are used as the definition of referable maculopathy which is termed M1 and should be referred to the hospital eye service (HES) for appropriate management or treatment. Patients with early macula changes will often be asymptomatic, thus stressing the importance of regular and accurate retinopathy screening.

Box 6.1 The NSC workbook (August 2007) stipulates that the best surrogate markers for predicting the presence of macula oedema and hence referable maculopathy includes

- Any exudate within 1DD of the fovea
- Circinate/tracking within 2DD of the fovea
- Retinal thickening within 1DD of the fovea (if stereo view available)
- Microaneurysm/haemorrhages within 1DD with best corrected VA of 6/12 or worse.

6.2 Classification of diabetic maculopathies

Maculopathy can occur in stages from early maculopathy to end-stage cystoid maculopathy. The three main forms of diabetic macular disease are exudative, ischaemic, and cystoid maculopathy, although there may be a mixed variety, commonly of ischaemic and exudative features.

6.2.1 Early maculopathy

Grading tools which allow manipulation and magnification of images may pick up possible early maculopathy. This may be presented as very subtle pale areas within the macula, representing possible early lipid leakage. More commonly, on magnification, digital images highlight areas of the macula with microaneurysms as a pale circular rim surrounding the microaneurysm which may signify early exudate leakage (Figure 6.2). Identification of possible early lipid leakage within 1DD of the fovea in the macula may present as early clinical signs of maculopathy. This should be graded M1 and referred for a clinical opinion to allow possible earlier intervention or monitoring. Poor VA of 6/12 or worse accompanied by microaneurysms or haemorrhages within the macula may also indicate early signs of significant maculopathy and should be graded M1 (Figure 6.3 and an example of macula microaneurysms in Appendix A2).

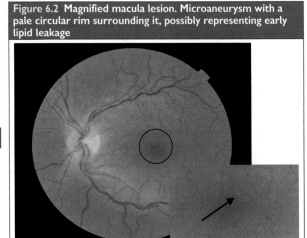

Figure 6.2 Magnified macula lesion. Microaneurysm with a pale circular rim surrounding it, possibly representing early lipid leakage

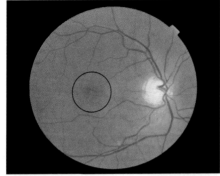

Figure 6.3 Early maculopathy. Clinical features of small microaneurysms located within 1DD of the fovea

6.2.2 Exudative maculopathy

Exudative maculopathy occurs due to the release of fats, proteins, and water from retinal capillaries. It is characterized by thick yellow waxy deposits of exudates with sharp finely defined borders which represent the residue of oedema. These types of retinal exudates tend to accumulate in the outer plexiform layer and may appear as discrete exudates within 1DD of the fovea (Figure 6.4). Any exudates within 1DD of the fovea should be graded as M1 and referred to HES for a routine appointment. However, if VA is affected an earlier appointment may be needed.

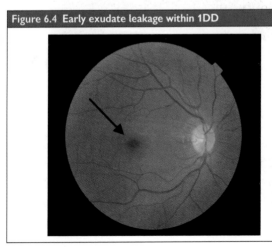

Figure 6.4 Early exudate leakage within 1DD

Exudates within the macula may also form certain patterns; the most common include a linear pattern of exudates known as tracking (streaks) into the fovea and a typical ring pattern known as a circinate.

6.2.3 Tracking exudates

Exudates within the macula may begin to impinge on the fovea; these exudates are derived from vessels in the macula area and are located between the radially arranged fibres of Henle's layer. This type of exudation is known as tracking (Figures 6.5) and may cause reduction in VA if it begins to encroach on the fovea. If poor VA accompanied by tracking exudates into the fovea is present, an earlier appointment to the HES is advised (within 6 weeks).

Figure 6.5 Characteristic appearance of tracking streaks of exudates temporal to the fovea

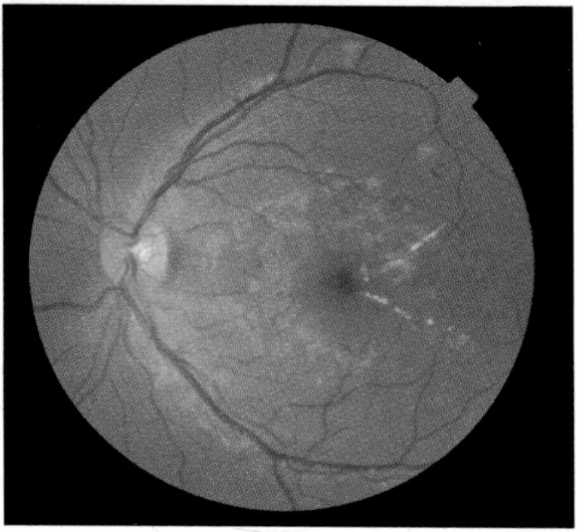

6.2.4 Circinate exudation

Exudates within 2DD of the fovea may also take on a ring-like or circinate form (Figure 6.6). The finely defined yellow thick deposits of lipid leakage conform around a retinal microaneurysm or capillary leakage.

Exudative maculopathy is further subdivided into *focal* and *diffuse* maculopathy which are characterized by the area of exudate and oedema within the macula.

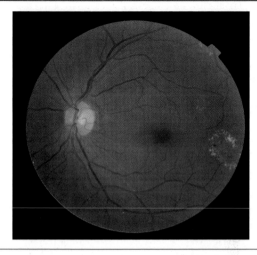

Figure 6.6 Circinate of exudates within 2DD temporal to the macula (edge of the image)

6.2.5 **Focal maculopathy**

Focal maculopathy is characterized by the distribution of exudates throughout the posterior pole. Exudates form in a ring shape/circinate focusing on one part of the macula region (Figure 6.7). Focal exudation is more commonly seen in the temporal region of the macula; this is known as the watershed area. Vision only becomes affected when the exudates begin to encroach upon the fovea. If clinically significant macula oedema (CSMO) is present in this area it may be treated by focal photocoagulation, and has the best response to focal laser treatment (see Chapter 17).

6.2.6 **Diffuse maculopathy**

Diffuse maculopathy occurs when exudates surround the whole macula (Figure 6.8), and is a more advanced disease with diffuse macula oedema and consequent visual loss. Grid laser may be used to treat this type of maculopathy, but the response to laser treatment is more limited than that to focal treatment (see Chapter 17).

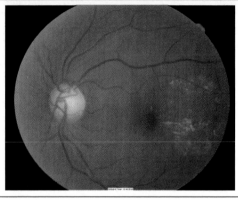

Figure 6.7 Focal maculopathy. The fundus images demonstrate how exudates are concentrated in one area on the macula and how they begin to impinge into the fovea

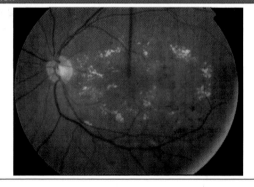

Figure 6.8 Diffuse maculopathy. Characteristic appearance of diffuse oedema and exudation affecting the whole macula region

6.2.7 Ischaemic maculopathy

Ischaemic maculopathy occurs due to hypoperfusion (retinal capillary closure) of the macula and requires urgent ophthalmology referral. It is characterized by a pale macula (due to deprived retinal circulation) accompanied by large blot strawberry haemorrhages, macula oedema, cotton wool spots, and reduced VA (Figure 6.9). Further investigations of retinal leakage/oedema are detected by fundus fluorescein angiograms or slit lamp biomicroscopy, highlighting areas of retinal thickening and ischaemia (see Chapter 17).

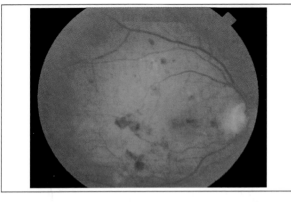

Figure 6.9 Ischaemic maculopathy. A distinctive fundus image of ischaemic maculopathy showing a pale macula and large red strawberry haemorrhages. There was macula oedema and 6/18 VA.

6.2.8 **Cystoid maculopathy**

Cystoid maculopathy occurs due to accumulation of extracellular fluid from the retinal capillaries into the macula area, causing retinal thickening. This indicates a breakdown of the inner blood-retinal barrier. It is characterized by a significant reduction in central vision and multiple petals around the macula representing cysts full of fluid (see Figure 6.10). Cystoid changes associated with diffuse or focal maculopathy frequently have a poorer prognosis and a disappointing response to photocoagulation, which can lead to irreversible loss of vision (see Chapter 17). This type of maculopathy requires urgent referral to the HES.

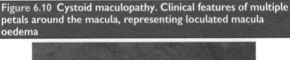

Figure 6.10 Cystoid maculopathy. Clinical features of multiple petals around the macula, representing loculated macula oedema

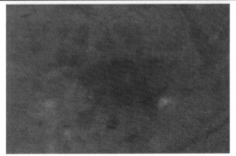

Table 6.1 Classification of diabetic maculopathy			
Types of macula disease	Clinical Features	Diabetic Maculopathy Grade	Outcome
Exudative (Focal)	Exudates concentrated in one area of the macula	M1	Routine ophthalmology referral
Exudative (Diffused)	Exudates surrounding the macula	M1	Routine ophthalmology referral
Ischaemic Maculopathy	Pale macula, cotton wool spots, and large blot (strawberry) haemorrhages	M1	Urgent ophthalmology referral
Cystoid Maculopathy	Retinal thickening and characteristic petals	M1	Urgent ophthalmology referral

Summary

Diabetic maculopathy needs referral to an ophthalmologist. According to the NSC guidelines, all referrals for maculopathy (M1) should be referred with a minimum standard of 70% < 13 weeks and an achievable standard of 95% < 13 weeks. The different types and features of maculopathy are summarized in Table 6.1.

Careful and regular accurate retinal screening is essential to detect early asymptomatic diabetic maculopathy, such that early and timely laser treatment can be applied, thereby preventing avoidable visual loss.

Further reading

Brownlee M (2001). Biochemistry and molecular cell biology of diabetic complications. *Nature,* **414**: 813–6.

Cook HL, Newsom R, Long V, Smith SA, Shilling JS, Stanford MR (1999). Natural history of diabetic macular streak exudates: evidence from a screening programme. *British Journal of Ophthalmology,* **83**: 563–6.

Dodson PM, Gibson JM, Kritzinger EE (1995). *Clinical retinopathies.* Chapman and Hall Medical 1st edition, London.

UK National Screening Committee (August 2007). Essential elements in developing a diabetic retinopathy screening programme; Workbook **4**: section 1.5.

Zander E, Herfurth S, Bohl B, Heinke P, Herrman U, Kohnert KD and Kerner W (2000). Maculopathy in patients with diabetes mellitus type 1 and type 2: associations with risk factors. *British Journal of Ophthalmology,* **84**: 871–6.

Chapter 7

Pre-proliferative and proliferative retinopathy

Rebecca Leigh

> **Key points**
>
> - Pre-proliferative retinopathy precedes proliferative retinopathy (new vessel growth) and is therefore an indication that the eye will soon be affected by advanced stages of retinopathy
> - Pre-proliferative retinopathy indicates chronic retinal ischaemia due to blocked capillaries and the clinical signs include
>   - Multiple cotton wool spots
>   - Venous beading and/or looping
>   - Multiple deep round and blot haemorrhages
>   - Intra-retinal microvascular abnormalities.
> - New vessels arise on the optic disc (NVD) or on the retinal surface (NVE) due to retinal ischaemia and growth factors (VEGF and others). The new vessels help re-vascularize the hypoxic (oxygen-starved) tissue.
> - New vessels can easily rupture, leading to haemorrhage and severe visual loss.

7.1 Pre-proliferative retinopathy

Pre-proliferative retinopathy is a clinically identifiable stage of diabetic retinopathy (DR). It is extremely important to recognize pre-proliferative retinopathy with its retinal signs, given that it precedes proliferative retinopathy (new vessel formation).

Background retinopathy is the earliest stage of DR and is characterized by
- Capillary wall thickening
- Pericyte loss
- Increased leukocyte adhesion to the vessel wall
- Alteration in blood flow.

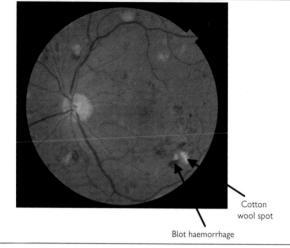

Figure 7.1 A fundus photograph showing a retina with pre-proliferative retinopathy. Cotton wool spots and blot haemorrhages are indicated

Cotton wool spot

Blot haemorrhage

As the disease progresses the retinal vessels become increasingly damaged, leading to progressive endothelial cell loss which in turn results in the occlusion of retinal capillaries and formation of extensive chronic retinal ischaemic areas. This is known as pre-proliferative retinopathy.

The clinical signs of pre-proliferative retinopathy (see Figure 7.1) that the screener/grader will be presented with include

- Cotton wool spots (Figure 7.2)
- Large blot haemorrhages (Figure 7.3)
- Intra-retinal microvascular abnormalities (IRMAs) (Figure 7.4)
- Venous abnormalities—beading (Figure 7.5), venous re-duplication (Figure 7.6), and venous loops.

7.1.1 Multiple cotton wool spots

Multiple cotton wool spots (Figure 7.2) are an important sign of advancing retinopathy and are an indication of retinal ischaemia. They are seen as greyish-white patches on the retina with feathery margins. However, they tend to change in appearance over months, forming pale areas of retina and losing their fluffy margins.

Cotton wool spots are produced by a blockage/reduced flow in a capillary resulting in the disruption of axoplasmic flow (the transport of molecules along a nerve cell axon) within the nerve fibre layers.

Figure 7.2 Example of a recent or fresh cotton wool spot

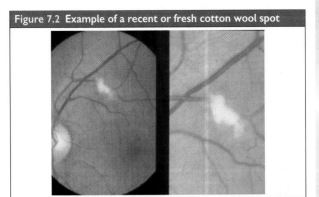

Figure 7.3 Example of a blot haemorrhage

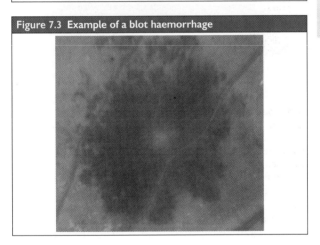

This in turn causes the neural tissue adjacent to the capillary occlusion to swell. Clinically they are described as focal ischaemic infarcts in the nerve fibre layer.

7.1.2 **Multiple deep round blot haemorrhages**

These are haemorrhages seen to be large and dark with a blot-like appearance, and often referred to as strawberry- or raspberry-shaped haemorrhages. They have irregular and indistinct borders. They are more sinister than dot haemorrhages because they occur in the deep layers of the retina and indicate retinal ischaemia (Figure 7.3).

7.1.3 **Intra-retinal microvascular abnormalities (IRMAs)**

These are areas of capillary dilatation and intra-retinal new vessel formation (i.e. vessels formed within the retina). They tend to form adjacent to or surround areas of occluded capillaries. They can sometimes be mistaken for new vessels on the surface of the retina. The definitve test to differentiate between each type is by fluorescein angiography (a technique for examining the circulation of the retina using the dye tracing method) as IRMAs do not leak. The presence of IRMAs within a retina is a definite indication of advanced pre-proliferative retinopathy (see Figure 7.4).

Figure 7.4 Example of IRMA

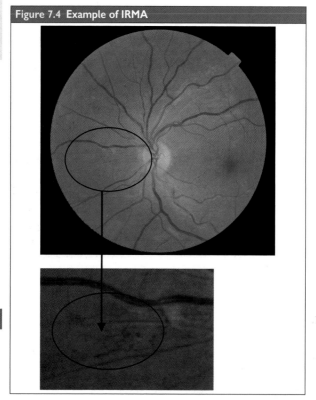

Figure 7.5 Venous irregularities and beading

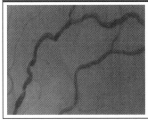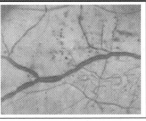

Figure 7.6 Venous reduplication and loops

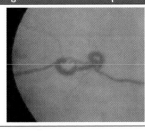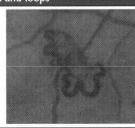

7.1.4 **Venous abnormalities**

Venous abnormalities occur as retinal ischaemia progresses and these abnormalities always signify serious retinal ischaemia with high and imminent risk of new vessel formation. These include venous beading and venous loops, as illustrated in Figures 7.5 and 7.6.

Venous beading is seen as irregular constriction and dilation of the lumen (inner space of vessel) of retinal venules. It occurs due to hypoxia which arises when there is extensive capillary occlusion and ischaemia. Initially the veins may show focal areas of dilation, but as the retinopathy progresses it may lead to significant venous beading and formation of venous loops/reduplication.

7.2 **Characterization of pre-proliferative retinopathy—NSC guidelines**

63

The National Screening Committee (NSC) guidelines for grading pre-proliferative retinopathy are as follows.

Pre-proliferative retinopathy (R2):

- Multiple deep, round or blot haemorrhages
- Venous beading

- Venous loop or re-duplication
- IRMAs
- The Birmingham Scheme includes >5 cotton wool spots in a retina.

More exact criteria for the definition are currently being considered e.g. what number of deep haemorrhages constitutes pre-proliferative rather than background changes. If the patient has the features of R2, a routine referral to ophthalmology is required as the risk of developing proliferative retinopathy is at least 50% over 2 years of follow-up. The principle is for patients with pre-proliferative retinopathy to be followed up by ophthalmologists so that laser treatment can be applied early owing to subsequent development of new vessels (proliferative retinopathy).

The NSC standards for referral for pre-proliferative retinopathy are as follows:

- *Achievable standard*: 95% to be seen by an ophthalmologist within less than 13 weeks
- *Minimum standard*: 70% to be seen within 13 weeks.

7.2.1 Pre-proliferative retinopathy and vision

Most patients with pre-proliferative diabetic retinopathy do not have visual symptoms, hence the importance of screening to detect this stage of disease. However, it has been reported that areas of significant retinal ischaemia correlate closely, although not always, to areas of reduced retinal sensitivity and hence visual field loss. The severity of the field loss has been shown to be variable especially with age, with less severe visual field loss in younger patients.

7.3 Proliferative retinopathy

The development of new vessels of the optic disc (NVD), on the surface of the retina (new vessels elsewhere, NVE) or on the iris, denotes the change from pre-proliferative retinopathy to the serious form of proliferative retinopathy. New vessels arise from retinal ischaemia and are presumed to be an attempt of revascularization of hypoxic tissue. The short- and the long-term consequences of new vessel formation are serious and affected patients have a high risk of suffering severe visual loss within 2 years. The significance of the new vessels is that they grow in the vitreo-retinal interface between the vitreous gel and retina with no support from surrounding structures. As their vessel walls are fragile they may fracture; hence a rupture results in pre-retinal (in front of the retina) and vitreous haemorrhage. If advanced, new vessels may also grow on the iris, called iris neovascularization, which in time may lead to intractable glaucoma which carries a poor visual prognosis (see Chapters 4 and 8).

7.3.1 **Pathogenesis**

The stimulus for pre-retinal new vessel growth is thought to be retinal hypoxia, caused by chronic retinal ischaemia, which in turn stimulates the release of vascular endothelial growth factor (VEGF). This protein is a primary mediator of retinal angiogenesis (the growth of new blood vessels from pre-existing vasculature).

VEGF was first discovered as a vascular permeability factor, but subsequently recognized as an angiogenic factor and as a specific mitogen (a protein that triggers cells to undertake cell division) for vascular endothelial cells. Its mRNA and proteins are expressed in retinal cell types including pericytes, astrocytes, glial cells, retinal pigment epithelial cells, and endothelial cells. It is released by these cells in response to hypoxia and binds with high affinity VEGF receptors expressed on vascular endothelial cells at the edge of the ischaemic area. This sets off a signalling cascade that affects the survival, proliferation, and migration of endothelial cells, eventually leading to new vessel growth. In animal experiments, injection of VEGF into the vitreous can induce pre-retinal and iris neovascularization.

A study demonstrating VEGF levels using immunostaining techniques has shown that VEGF is absent or in low levels in the majority of normal retinas. The VEGF level increases with pre-proliferative retinopathy, as the staining is of greater intensity, and it is shown to be highly elevated in diabetic patients with active proliferative retinopathy with intense staining in the retinal vessels, the choroid, and the ganglion cell layer.

It has been shown, however, that VEGF inhibition alone is insufficient to prevent retinal neovascularization. It has therefore been suggested that there are other mediators of retinal angiogenesis, examples including growth hormone (GH), insulin-like growth factor-1 (IGF-1), angiotensins, erythropoietin, and fibroblast growth factor (FGF) (see Chapter 16).

7.3.2 **Retinal signs**

The clinical signs of proliferative retinopathy are new vessels either on the retina (new vessels elsewhere, NVE) or on the optic disc (new vessels on the optic disc, NVD) (Figure 7.7), arising from the venous side of the circulation.

NVE occur away from the optic disc in the vascular arcades above and below the macula and in the watershed areas temporal to the macula. However, they can occur in the nasal area and these can be easily missed. They invariably develop from the veins adjacent to areas of retinal ischaemia, arising in lacy networks of radiating spokes from vessels. They often cross over both the arteries and veins in the retina, indicating unregulated growth. Due to their fine calibre they may be easily missed. Untreated NVE in particular are associated with retinal detachment, hence the importance of their early detection and treatment. If identified, *de novo*, patients should have an urgent referral as they can either remain relatively stable or grow rapidly and bleed (Figure 7.8).

Figure 7.7 Showing **NVD** and superiorly **NVE** with gliosis

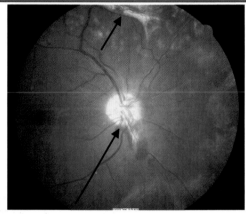

New vessels on the optic disc (NVD). Note pan retinal photocoagulation visible in peripheral nasal region.

Figure 7.8 Proliferative retinopathy showing signs of **NVE**

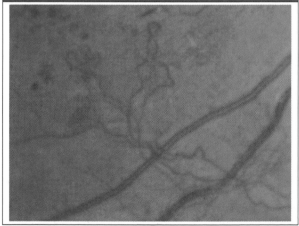

Figure 7.9 New vessels on the optic disc (NVD)

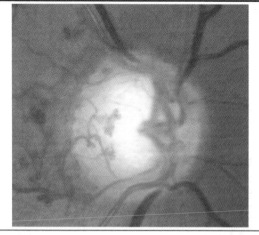

New vessels occurring on the optic disc or within one diameter of the optic disc should be referred urgently as they are particularly threatening to vision, as they carry a high risk of vitreous haemorrhage, if allowed to progress (Figure 7.9).

7.3.3 **NSC Guidelines**

The NSC guidelines for grading proliferative retinopathy are as follows:
Proliferative retinopathy (R3):

- New vessels elsewhere (NVE)
- New vessels on the disc (NVD)
- Pre-retinal/vitreous haemorrhage (see Chapter 8, section 8.2 and 8.3).

If the patient has the features of R3, an urgent referral to ophthalmology is required as there is a high risk of vitreous haemorrhage and development of advanced sight-threatening retinopathy.

The NSC standards for referral of new vessels state the following:

- *Achievable standard*: 95% to be seen by an ophthalmologist within 2 weeks from date of screen
- *Minimum standard*: 70% to be seen within 2 weeks.

The severity of proliferative retinopathy can be classified by the presence or absence of high risk characteristics for visual loss. The Diabetic Retinopathy Study (DRS) and Early Treatment Diabetic Retinopathy Study (ETDRS) determined the high-risk characteristics.

If an eye has three of the following four characteristics it is deemed as high risk:

- Presence of any neovascularization
- Neovascularization on or within 1DD of the optic disc
- A moderate to severe amount of neovascularization (greater than one-third of a disc area, or new vessels elsewhere greater than half a disc area)
- Vitreous haemorrhage.

If untreated, 26% of eyes with 'high risk' and NVD will progress to severe visual loss within 2 years. With laser treatment this figure is reduced to 11% (see Chapter 17).

Summary

Pre-proliferative retinopathy heralds the development of more sinister proliferative changes which may threaten vision. Referral should be made through to ophthalmology clinics so these patients can be followed up by accurate slit lamp bio-microscopy to pick early proliferative changes. The new finding of proliferative retinopathy in a diabetic patient is an urgent referral to eye services as pre-retinal and vitreous haemorrhage may be imminent; the latter may obscure the retinal view for many months, preventing laser treatment. Before the digital camera screening programme, a UK national audit of referrals to diabetic eye clinics indicated that 25% of patients with proliferative retinopathy were presenting at a late stage with visual symptoms (due to haemorrhage). This reinforces the importance of accurate retinal screening.

Further reading

Boulton M, Foreman D, *et al.* (1998). VEGF localisation in diabetic retinopathy. *British Journal of Ophthalmology,* **82**: 561–8.

Caroline K Chee and Declan W Flanagan (1993). Visual field loss with capillary non-perfusion in preproliferative and early proliferative diabetic retinopathy. *British Journal of Ophthalmology;* **77**: 726–30.

Kohner EM (1993). Diabetic retinopathy. *British Medical Journal,* **307**: 1195–9.

Livingstone C and Ferns G (2003). Insulin-like growth factor-related proteins and diabetic complications. *The British Journal of Diabetes and Vascular Disease,* **3**(5): 326–9.

Mitamura Y and Harada C (2005). Role of cytokines and trophic factors in the pathogenesis of diabetic retinopathy. *Current Diabetes Reviews*, **1**: 73–81.

Schultz GS and Grant MB (1991). Neovascular growth factors. *Eye*, **5**: 170–80.

Watanabe D, Suzuma K, Matsui S, Kurimoto M, Kiryu J, Kita M. (2005). Erythropoietin as a retinal angiogenic factor in proliferative diabetic retinopathy. *The New England Journal of Medicine*, **353**: 782–92.

Chapter 8

Advanced diabetic eye disease

Karen Whitehouse

> **Key points**
>
> - Hypoxia of the retina leads to development of new vessels which subsequently may form fibrous and glial tissue.
> - Gliosis and fibrosis in the new vessels from the retina onto the posterior vitreous interface may cause retinal traction and retinal detachment.
> - New blood vessels can also grow into the angle of the anterior chamber of the eye (rubeosis iridis) leading to neovascular or rubeotic glaucoma.
> - Rubeotic glaucoma is a serious complication with visual loss and raised intra-ocular pressure, resulting eventually in acute severe periorbital pain, corneal oedema, and optic atrophy.
> - Advanced diabetic eye disease can remain asymptomatic for a long time, due to the slow progression of proliferative retinopathy.
> - Diabetic retinopathy screening is an important factor in early identification and following timely laser, may prevent development of advanced disease.

8.1 Introduction

Advanced diabetic eye disease may be classed as end-stage damage from diabetic retinopathy (DR), causes permanent visual impairment and blindness among diabetic adults. Both type 1 and type 2 patients are at risk. Hyperglycaemia-induced microvascular complications of diabetes include increased vascular permeability, ischaemia, and formation of new vessels (neovascularization). Neovascularization of the retina generates a high risk of vitreous haemorrhage and fibrosis.

The leading cause of persistent severe visual loss in proliferative DR is vitreous or pre-retinal haemorrhage, followed by macular oedema/pigmentary changes associated with macular oedema. The third is due to retinal detachment. The incidence of severe visual loss can be reduced with photocoagulation and vitrectomy surgery. These processes will now be outlined.

Box 8.1 NSC Standards for Referral

The English National Screening Programme for Diabetic Retinopathy benchmark standards state that referral of advanced stage conditions are as follows:

Achievable standard: 95 % seen by ophthalmologist within 1 week
Minimum standard: 70% seen by ophthalmologist within 1 week
100% seen by ophthalmologist within 2 weeks

Our policy is that patients presenting with sudden loss of vision or suspicion of rubeotic glaucoma should be seen urgently in an eye casualty department, or, if seen during a hospital DR screening clinic, to the Hospital Eye Service.

The aim of regular and accurate retinal screening is to avoid development of advanced DR changes. Patients, however, still present to our DR screening service for the first time with advanced disease, sadly often too late for restoration of vision.

8.2 Subhyaloid/pre-retinal haemorrhage

Widespread retinal ischaemia stimulates the formation of new vessels which arise from the retinal venous circulation in a characteristic pattern, forming loops or a fine meshwork. New vessels either form on the optic disc (NVD) or in the peripheral retina (NVE). The new vessels grow forwards on to the posterior vitreous interface and subsequently into the vitreous gel. Whilst the vitreous humour is a transparent gel filling, it is a mobile structure such that the delicate new vessels are disrupted by movement and traction within the vitreous, which will cause the fragile new vessels to bleed. The haemorrhage occurs either in the level of subhyaloid space between posterior vitreous face and retina or under the internal limiting membrane, resulting in either pre-retinal or subhyaloid haemorrhage (Figures 8.1 and 8.2).

As haemorrhage forms, it takes on a characteristic appearance with a fluid level due to gravity (Figure 8.1). The patient may complain of floaters or 'spots' in the vision, but may present with severe visual loss if the haemorrhage is anterior and covering the macula area. Any new appearance of pre-retinal or subhyaloid haemorrhage is a serious complication and the screener/grader will grade this as R3 (as in proliferative retinopathy) with a recommendation for urgent

Figure 8.1 Boat-shaped haemorrhage from new vessels on the optic disc (NVD)–a pre-retinal haemorrhage

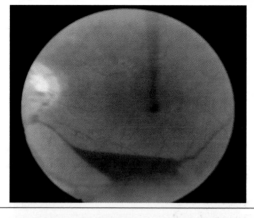

Figure 8.2 Diabetic patient presenting with blurred vision. Haemorrhage has occurred between the retinal surface and the hyaloid face of the vitreous–a subhyaloid haemorrhage

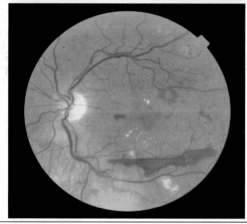

referral, as per NSC standards. The reason for the urgency is that further haemorrhage may break through into the vitreous cavity producing a vitreous haemorrhage. This may produce a visual disaster as the patient cannot see and the ophthalmologist cannot obtain a retinal view.

8.3 Vitreous haemorrhage

Between 31% and 54% of vitreous haemorrhages are due to DR. Sight-threatening vitreous haemorrhage occurs abruptly and painlessly. In early haemorrhage, the patients will complain of a sudden onset of floaters or a cobweb image across their vision or the vision may become reddened and hazy. However, severe or advanced haemorrhage can compromise visual acuity (VA) dramatically, causing areas of diminished sight within the visual field (scotomas) or profound visual loss. The patient may note that the vision is worse when lying in a prone position, due to haemorrhage shifting within the vitreous and obscuring the macula (see Figure 8.3).

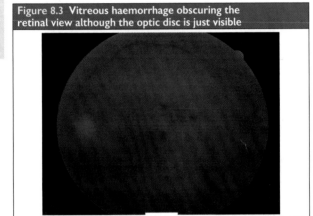

Figure 8.3 Vitreous haemorrhage obscuring the retinal view although the optic disc is just visible

The screener/grader may be presented with a red haze obscuring the retinal blood vessels and/or the optic nerve, indicating a less severe haemorrhage, or a dense red fundus with indistinct detail of retinal blood vessels and optic nerve, which indicates a severe vitreous haemorrhage (Figure 8.3). All cases of vitreous haemorrhage will be graded as R3—urgent referral—and should be seen in either an eye casualty or must be directed to a hospital for an emergency ophthalmological assessment.

Vitreous haemorrhage slowly resolves at a rate of approximately 1% per day, clearing more quickly in vitrectomized eyes and more slowly in younger eyes. Vitreous haemorrhage does, however, take many months to resolve. In a number of cases though, the underlying proliferative retinopathy may lead to further repeated haemorrhages, such that vision does not improve and retinal examination is still not possible. This is one of the major indications for vitrectomy surgery.

8.4 **Gliosis**

As the disease develops further, the process of neovascularization causes scarring (gliosis), as fibrous tissue develops around the new vessels. The fibrous tissue may eventually contract, and with traction develop into tractional retinal detachment. This will give the appearance of fibrous strands emanating in the new vessel glial complex; once the gliotic membrane is large, it is immobile (Figures 8.4 and 8.5).

Figure 8.4 Extensive gliosis of NVD, resulting in traction of the superior temporal arcade, and obliterating both the macula and optic disc

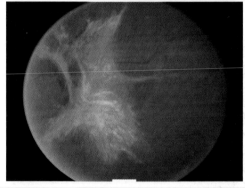

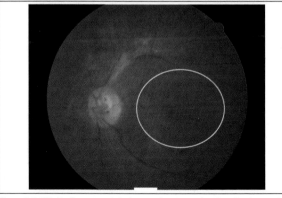

Figure 8.5 Gliosis of new vessels in the superior temporal and nasal retina resulting in an epiretinal membrane (ERM) formation of the macula (circled)—notice the typical puckering and lines of the ERM in the macula region.

8.5 **Tractional retinal detachment**

Proliferative DR is the primary causative factor in tractional retinal detachments. The gliosis resulting from new vessels may contract and subsequently pull the retina from the underlying retinal pigment epithelium (RPE). Studies suggest that soluble vascular cell adhesion molecules may contribute to progression of neovascularization and fibrosis as a result of endothelial, Müller, and retinal pigment epithelial cell activation. Retinal detachment also augments the existing inflammation within the diabetic retina.

Tractional retinal detachments develop slowly, progressing as fibrovascular proliferation increases. Peripheral tractional detachments are therefore rarely, if ever, noticed by the patient. Macular tractional detachments, on the other hand, tend to be symptomatic, as VA will be affected. The patient may complain of a veiled effect or 'curtain' across their field of vision; if the macula is affected they may notice that straight lines appear distorted. The highest elevation of the retina occurs at the traction site and vessels are pulled towards the adhesions (Figures 8.6 and 8.7). Traction on the macula requires an urgent vitrectomy specialist opinion.

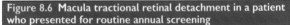

Figure 8.6 Macula tractional retinal detachment in a patient who presented for routine annual screening

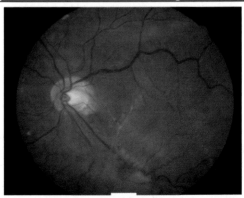

Figure 8.7 Tractional retinal detachment at the optic disc

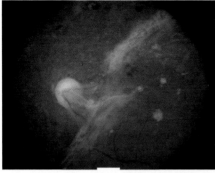

Figure 8.8 New vessels growing on the pupillary margin—rubeosis iridis

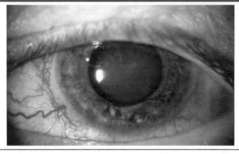

8.6 Iris new vessels—rubeosis iridis—rubeotic glaucoma

In cases of advanced proliferative retinopathy, vascular proliferation may extend into the posterior iris, through the pupil, along the anterior surface of the iris (Figure 8.8), and into the Canal of Schlemm, thereby reducing drainage of aqueous humour. This produces acute glaucoma with markedly raised intra-ocular pressure, periorbital pain, and visual loss; the patient will complain of an intensely painful eye. This in turn causes the cornea to become oedematous, and the optic nerve, affected by the high intra-ocular pressure, becomes atrophic. If the disease develops, the fibrous membrane contracts causing synaechiae—adhesion of the iris to the cornea or of the iris to the lens. This is an emergency clinical situation and patients need to be seen in an eye casualty for assessment, analgesia, and treatment of raised intra-ocular pressure.

Further reading

Astrid Limb G, Hickman-Casey J, Hollifield RD, and Chignell AH. (1999). Vascular adhesion molecules in vitreous from eyes with proliferative diabetic retinopathy. *Investigative Ophthalmology and Visual Science*, **40**: 2453–7.

Berdahl JP and Mruthyunjaya P. In Ingrid U. Scott and Sharon Fekrat eds. *Vitreous hemorrhage: diagnosis and treatment*. American Academy Ophthalmology Publications.

Fong DS, Ferris FL 3rd, Davis MD, Chew EY (1999). Causes of severe visual loss in the early treatment diabetic retinopathy study: ETDRS report no. 24. *American Journal of Ophthalmology*, Feb; **127**(2): 137–41.

NDT Advance Access published online on November 22, 2006 Nephrology Dialysis Transplantation, doi:10.1093/ndt/gfl641.

Negi A and Vernon SA (2003). An overview of the eye in diabetes. *Journal of the Royal Society Medicine,* **96**: 266–72.

Nork TM, Wallow IH, Sramek SJ, Anderson G (1987). Müller's cell involvement in proliferative diabetic retinopathy. *Archives of Ophthalmology*, Oct; **105**(10): 1424–9.

Ray D, Mishra M, Ralph S, Read I, Davies R, Brenchley P (2004). Association of the VEGF gene with proliferative diabetic retinopathy but not Proteinuria in diabetes. *Diabetes*, **53**: 861–4.

Chapter 9

Other ophthalmic lesions in the fundus

Jonathan M Gibson

Key points

- When screening the diabetic population for diabetic retinopathy (DR), many other retinal conditions will be identified.
- The most common conditions which may be diagnosed as DR are retinal vein and artery occlusion, hypertensive retinopathy, arterial emboli, and retinal changes due to blood disorders, for example, anaemia. These need local protocols for medical management.
- Familiarity and pattern recognition are important to recognize common abnormalities, for example, drusen, chorioretinitis, asteroides hyalosis, choroidal naevi, and age-related macula degeneration.

9.1 Introduction

Retinal screening of patients with digital fundus photography throws up a number of images which are puzzling for the grader, and these may represent harmless variations of normality or serious ophthalmic pathology. In this chapter, examples of the common and important abnormalities that might be detected and details on what to do about them are given.

9.2 Retinal drusen

Retinal drusen are a common finding in elderly patients and represent age-related changes in Bruch's membrane, the basement membrane of the retinal pigment epithelium. They are, therefore, situated under the retina and appear as discrete yellowish lesions (see Figures 9.1 and 9.2).

The importance of drusen in the context of diabetic retinopathy (DR) lies in differentiating them from diabetic retinal exudates. They are a manifestation of age-related macular degeneration (AMD) and the soft types can predispose to the formation of choroidal neovascular membrane and the loss of central vision (Table 9.1).

Figure 9.1 Retinal drusen in typical appearance

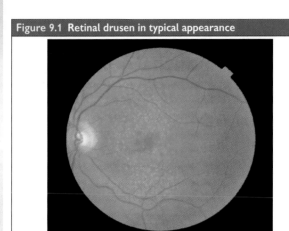

Figure 9.2 Red-free fundus photographs of right and left eyes in the same patient showing soft retinal drusen at the macula and the symmetrical position in each eye

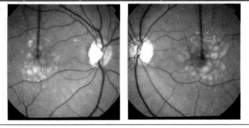

Table 9.1 Comparison of main features of retinal drusen and exudates

Criteria	Drusen	Exudates
Colour	Yellow	Creamy white
Edges	Tend to be soft	Tend to be hard
Symmetry between eyes	Always symmetrical	Occasionally symmetrical
Situation in fundus	Always at macula	Can be anywhere—often circinate
Which layer of retina	Subretinal	Intra-retinal

Patients in whom retinal drusen are detected on screening do not require referral to the eye clinic unless the patient is known to be suffering from visual symptoms, of which distortion of images is the most important.

9.3 Abnormalities of fundus pigmentation

Congenital pigmentation of the retina may occur as congenital hypertrophy of the retinal pigment epithelium (CHRPE) or as a characteristic bear track pigmentation, which looks like a trail of muddy footprints (Figure 9.3). These are both harmless findings although CHRPE, when in large numbers or bilateral, have been associated with familial polyposis coli in susceptible individuals.

Acquired pigmented lesions may occur from choroidal naevi and tumours, previous inflammatory disease of the choroid and retina, and from pre-existing laser scars (Figure 9.4).

Figure 9.3 **Bear track pigmentation in superotemporal quadrant**

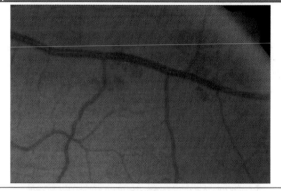

Figure 9.4 **Pigmentation from heavy macular laser photo-coagulation 10 years earlier**

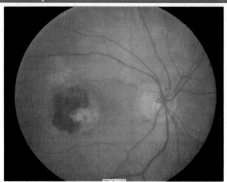

Choroidal naevi are a common finding in Caucasians and are estimated to occur in up to 30% of the population. They are benign melanocytic tumours but rarely may become malignant in 1 in 5000 cases. The main significance of choroidal naevi is to distinguish them from malignant melanoma of the choroid (Figure 9.5). Signs of malignant change in naevi may be subtle, but the following mnemonic can be helpful.

9.3.1 **TFSOM: 'To Find Small Ocular Melanomas'**

- Thickness (>2mm)
- Fluid (Subretinal)
- Symptoms
- Orange pigment (lipofuscin in the lesion)
- Margin touching disc (Shields 2002).

In the absence of any of the above features the lesion is unlikely to be a malignant melanoma. However, it may be difficult for the grader or screener to appreciate all the above features from two dimensional retinal photographs alone and, in general, it is advisable to gain advice on the policy of referral of suspicious lesions from the local ophthalmologists.

Management of choroidal naevi that are not suspicious is usually by means of serial fundus photography by the local referring optometrist or by the hospital eye department.

9.3.2 **Myelinated nerve fibres**

These occur when the normal process of myelination of the optic nerve continues beyond the lamina cribrosa into the retinal nerve fibres. They have a characteristic creamy white appearance (Figure 9.6) with a feathery margin at the peripheral part of the lesion and are generally a harmless finding, requiring no further investigation.

Figure 9.5 Choroidal naevi in separate patients. The lesion adjacent to the disc is suspicious and should be referred to the ophthalmology clinic

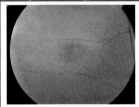 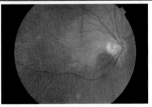

Figure 9.6 Myelinated nerve fibres

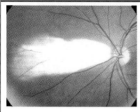 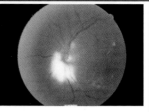

Figure 9.7 Fundus of a highly myopic patient showing peri-papillary atrophic and pigmentary changes, and a single lacquer crack extending inferior to the macula

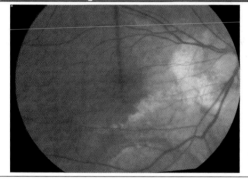

9.3.3 Myopia

There are a number of fundal appearances associated with myopia which are harmless. These range from pale areas of choroido-retinal atrophy around the optic disc, the so-called myopic crescent to areas of pale streaks corresponding to ruptures in Bruch's membrane, the basement membrane of the retina. These latter abnormalities are termed 'lacquer cracks' (Figure 9.7).

Occasionally the defects caused by the myopia can cause growth of subretinal blood vessels representing a choroidal neovascular membrane, and therefore any associated macular haemorrhage in myopic fundi should be treated with suspicion and referred to the ophthalmologists for tertiary grading or to the eye clinic.

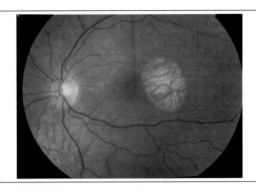

Figure 9.8 Laser photocoagulation scar from previous treatment for wet macular degeneration 5 years earlier. Atrophy of the retinal pigment epithelium shows visible underlying large choroidal blood vessels and sclera.

9.3.4 Laser photocoagulation scars

Laser photocoagulation reactions are seen immediately as greyish white discrete lesions, but within a few weeks pigmentary and atrophic changes start to become visible. Reactions may be predominantly atrophic or pigmented (Figures 9.4 and 9.8).

9.4 Inflammatory disease

Previous inactive choroiditis and retinitis scars are commonly seen in fundus photographs but it may be impossible to determine a cause, and in many cases they represent long-standing childhood or congenital lesions. Active inflammatory lesions are most unlikely to be detected by retinal screening for DR because patients would notice reduced vision and other symptoms. Signs of active inflammation are very hazy pictures, as a result of associated vitritis, and haemorrhage and fuzzy white, creamy lesions in the fundus. Suspected cases should be referred to the ophthalmologist for urgent investigation.

Toxoplasmosis is probably the most common infectious disease involving the retina and is caused by *Toxoplasma gondii*, a sporozoan parasite with a two-host life cycle. Congenital infection or acquired infection in immunocompromised individuals can be associated with retinal infection (a retinitis). Inactive healed lesions are the ones most likely to be found in retinopathy screening and the characteristic appearance is of a large, well-defined scar surrounded by pigment (Figures 9.9 and 9.10).

Common causes of inflammatory scars due to retinitis are toxoplasmosis, toxocariasis, syphilis, and herpes virus infections including cytomegalovirus. An important cause of choroidal infection is tuberculosis.

Figure 9.9 Single scar presumed to be due to congenital toxoplasmosis

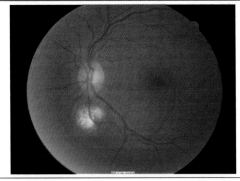

Figure 9.10 Fundus shows multifocal scars and subretinal fibrosis under fovea. Case of inactive multifocal choroiditis

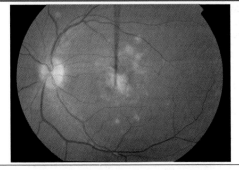

9.5 **Retinovascular disorders**

The commonest retinovascular disorders that are likely to be detected during screening photography are branch and central retinal vein occlusions and retinal artery macroaneurysms.

9.5.1 **Branch retinal vein occlusion**

Branch retinal vein occlusion (BRVO) occurs at crossing points where a retinal vein and arteriole share a common adventitial sheath. In most cases the arteriole is anterior to the corresponding vein and compression of the vein causes an occlusion. Cases are classified depending on the size of the vein occluded and can vary from a small occlusion affecting the macula to a whole quadrant of the fundus, the superotemporal being the most likely to be affected (Figure 9.11).

If the macula is involved, vision is invariably affected but the prognosis in the longer term depends on how much associated ischaemic damage occurs to the capillary circulation at the macula.

Clinical features are variable and patients may be asymptomatic if the macula is not involved. Haemorrhages are flame shaped, dot and blot, and in more severe cases, confluent and of a dark colour. Other findings are cotton wool spots and dilated retinal veins in the affected quadrant, exudates (chronic phase), pigment disturbance and collateral vessels may occur. Fluorescein angiography (FFA) may be useful in assessing which cases may require laser treatment.

Management of BRVO consists of investigation as to the cause and modification of any underlying medical risk factors, of which systemic hypertension is most common (see section 9.5.2). Ophthalmic treatment is indicated if there is macular oedema, visual acuity (VA) of 6/12 or worse, and no spontaneous improvement in 3–6 months. Macular grid laser treatment and intra-vitreal injections of anti-VEGF agents are the mainstay of treatment for macular oedema, and sectoral pan-retinal photocoagulation laser may be required for retinal neovascularization. About 50% of cases will spontaneously settle and achieve vision of 6/12 or better.

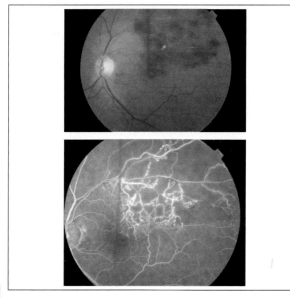

Figure 9.11 Superotemporal branch retinal vein occlusion on fundus photography and fluorescein angiogram, showing retinal haemorrhages and single cotton wool spot in the acute phase and associated capillary fall-out on angiography. Vision was 6/9.

9.5.2 **Central retinal vein occlusion**

Central retinal vein occlusions (CRVO) and hemi-CRVO (see Figures 9.12 and 9.13) occur when the central retinal vein is occluded posterior to the cribriform plate. They are classified clinically as ischaemic and non-ischaemic on the basis of fundus examination and fluorescein angiographic findings.

All patients with branch (BRVO) and CRVO require investigation, which should include blood pressure, full blood count, erythrocyte sedimentation ratio (ESR), urea and electrolytes, glucose, lipids, protein electrophoresis, thyroid function tests, and ECG. Patients should be referred for an ophthalmologist's opinion as soon as possible for investigation and possible treatment. Management of CRVO will depend on whether it is classified as ischaemic or non-ischaemic, and this is based on clinical examination and in some cases, fluorescein angiography.

It is important to treat any underlying medical conditions to prevent recurrence in the fellow eye and this is best achieved with the ophthalmologist liaising with a physician. Treatment options include management of raised intra-ocular pressure, laser panretinal photocoagulation (PRP), and intra-vitreal injection of anti-VEGF agents.

Figure 9.12 Superior, hemi-central retinal vein occlusion with haemorrhages and multiple cotton wool spots visible

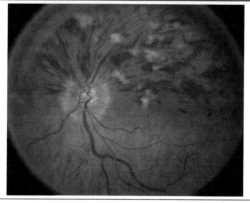

9.5.3 **Retinal arterial occlusion**

These are ophthalmic emergencies which present with sudden loss of vision (for examples, see Figure 4.2). They are most unlikely to present to the screening programme because of this and they require urgent medical care.

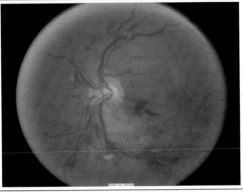

Figure 9.13 Non-ischaemic CRVO with haemorrhages in all four quadrants, cotton wool spots, and dilated veins

9.5.4 Retinal arteriolar emboli

Emboli in the retinal arterioles are a common finding in fundus photographs, and the majority are asymptomatic (see Figure 9.16). They may originate from the carotid arteries associated with athero-sclerosis or more rarely they may originate from the heart. The commonest appearance, the cholesterol embolus or Hollenhorst plaque, is of a highly refractile lesion within an arteriole commonly at a bifurcation in the vessel.

Patients in whom an embolus is detected should be referred to a physician for further medical investigation urgently in case the patient is at risk of cerebrovascular emboli and stroke. Diagnosis is made by the history and special investigations including Doppler scanning of the carotid arteries. Management involves reducing the risk of emboli being shed and may require a carotid endarterecomy being performed.

9.5.5 Hypertensive retinopathy

Systemic hypertension is one of the commonest diseases of the Western world and is commonly found in patients with diabetes mellitus. Ophthalmic features are focal narrowing and irregularity of the retinal arterioles, and in more severe cases cotton wool spots and retinal haemorrhages, both flame shaped in the nerve fibre layer and deeper blot haemorrhages (Figure 9.14). It should be noted that arterio-venous nipping or nicking is more usually considered a sign of arteriosclerotic disease, although this commonly coexists with hypertensive changes.

Accelerated hypertension (Figure 9.14) occurs when the blood pressure is severely raised, for example, >220mmHg systolic and >120mmHg diastolic pressures. Fundal features are as described before but with optic disc swelling and exudates in a star pattern at the macula. Patients in this category should be referred urgently.

The original classification of hypertensive retinopathy by Keith, Wagener, and Barker in 1939 was based on correlation of the fundus findings and the severity of hypertension and survival risk of the patient. More recent grading schemes have tried to recognize the modern change in survival rates of patients and have reflected this in simplified schemes (see Table 9.2).

Figure 9.14 Accelerated hypertension in a patient sent for DR screening and with BP of 230/140mmHg

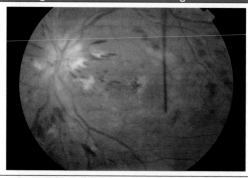

Table 9.2 Grading for hypertensive retinopathy

Grade	Retinal changes	Hypertension severity	Prognosis
A	Arteriolar narrowing, focal constriction	Non-malignant	Depends on BP, age, other risk factors, and end-organ damage
B	Haemorrhages, exudates C/W spots ± papillodaema	Accelerated/ malignant	80% dead in 2 years if not treated. Prognosis depends on BP control

9.5.6 **Macroaneurysms**

Retinal arteriolar macroaneurysms are focal dilatations of retinal arterioles and are much larger than microaneurysms, usually 100–250mcm in size. They are often asymptomatic but vision can be threatened by slow exudative decompensation of the lesion which can threaten the macula or from acute haemorrhage (Figure 9.15). Haemorrhage from macroaneurysms is unusual in that it can occur in subretinal, intra-retinal, and pre-retinal planes as well as breaking through into the vitreous.

Macroaneurysms are associated most commonly with systemic hypertension but may also be associated with carotid artery disease, and patients in whom asymptomatic lesions are found should be referred to a physician for further investigation.

In most cases, spontaneous resolution occurs but if the vision is threatened retinal focal laser photocoagulation either directly to seal off the macroaneurysm or indirectly around the lesion can be performed.

Figure 9.15 Two retinal arteriolar macroaneurysms arising from the same retinal vessel

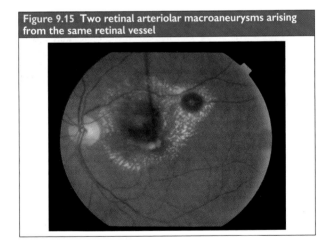

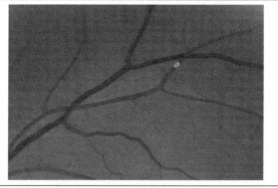

Figure 9.16 A yellow refractive lesion is seen at the arteriolar bifurcation–a cholestrol embolus

9.6 **Rarer abnormalities**

Anomalous vascular patterns in the retina may occur with vessels encroaching and crossing the macular region and crossing the horizontal raphe (the imaginary continued line from the optic disc to the fovea). These abnormal vascular patterns are usually congenital and asymptomatic although the abnormal vessels are more likely to develop pathological changes, presumably due to abnormal blood flow.

9.6.1 **Retinal detachment** (Figure 9.17)

These are usually symptomatic and would usually present as an emergency to the ophthalmic department with loss of vision. If the macula is attached, however, central vision will be unaffected and patients may be unaware.

9.6.2 **Asteroides hyalosis** (Figure 9.18)

This unusual condition, which is caused by degenerative changes in the vitreous gel, gives the appearance of multiple reflective floaters in front of the retina. If the condition is marked as in the example given here, fundus photography may not be able to show the retina clearly. In most cases, this is a harmless asymptomatic condition but if photography is poor they should be referred to the eye clinic for examination.

Figure 9.17 Bullous retinal detachment with a large area of serous retinal detachment

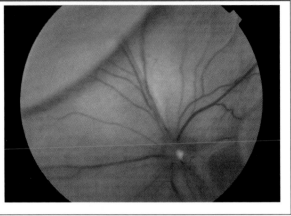

Figure 9.18 A case of asteroides hyalosis with poor retinal visualization that required referral to the eye clinic for annual DR screening

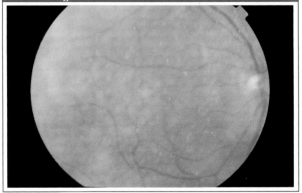

Further reading

Denniston AKO and Murray PI (2006). *Oxford handbook of ophthalmology.* Oxford University Press, Oxford.

Dodson PM, Gibson JM, Kritzinger EE (1994). *Clinical retinopathies.* Hodder Headline, London.

Shields CL, Shields JA (2002). Clinical features of small choroidal melanoma. *Current Opinion in Ophthalmology,* **13**: 135–141.

Chapter 10

The screening episode—visual acuity, mydriasis, and digital photography

David Roy and Jane Pitt

> ### Key points
>
> - Digital retinal photography has completely revolutionized the accurate detection of diabetic retinopathy (DR), allowing precise diagnosis and resulting in timely and appropriate referral to diabetic eye specialists.
> - Accurate measurement of visual acuity (VA) followed by adequate pupil dilatation (mydriasis) is an integral part of a DR screening episode.
> - A visual history is essential to record, as this may affect the clinical outcome of screening.
> - Obtaining digital retinal photographs (images) of acceptable quality to grade, with a low ungradable rate (< 10%), is imperative.
> - Practice and expertise is needed to ensure avoidance of the pitfalls of digital photography.

10.1 Measuring visual acuity/drop instillation

10.1.1 Visual acuity

Visual 'acuity' (VA) is derived from the latin word *acuitas* (sharpness). It is used to describe the smallest letters which can be read without refractive correction on a visual acuity chart.

A common method for measuring VA is using the Snellen chart (see Figure 10.1) devised by a Dutch ophthalmologist Dr Herman Snellen in 1892. The chart consists of 11 lines of printed block letters. The first line consists of the largest letter, which may be one of several letters, followed by rows of letters decreasing in size.

A person taking the test covers one eye and reads aloud the letters of each row, starting from the top. The smallest letter row that can be read accurately indicates the patient's VA in that eye, and is recorded. This is then repeated using methods to correct refractive error (e.g. glasses and/or pin hole test). More recently, healthcare professionals are introducing the Logmar chart (logarithm of the minimum angle of resolution) (see Figure 10.2) following recommendations of the American National Academy of Sciences National Research Council. The Logmar method has been found to be more accurate and reproducible than the Snellen method, and is being introduced into routine clinical practice.

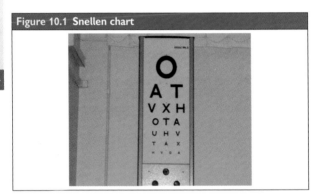

Figure 10.1 Snellen chart

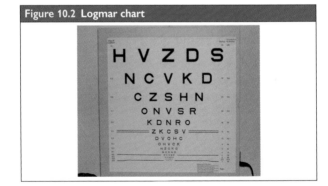

Figure 10.2 Logmar chart

10.2 **VA testing during a screening episode**

10.2.1 **The importance of VA testing**

Visual acuity (VA) is the most important measurement of visual function and should be measured with the patient wearing their glasses to correct known refractive error. Alternatively or as well as, the simple pinhole device may be used, which only allows light rays through the principal axis to the retina thus minimizes refractive errors of the cornea and lens and, therefore, provides a measure of best corrected vision. At every screening episode, patients with diabetes should have their VA measured and recorded on the screening software as it is also integral to the clinical outcome, for example, the referable maculopathy definition outlined in Chapter 6. Where previous screening information and VA are available it is also a useful comparison to assess change which could indicate ocular disease.

The retinal screener, following measurement of the VA, should enquire on the nature and timings of visual loss, as well previous ocular interventions and record the details. For example, a patient with uniocular poor vision may be the result of amblyopia, commonly as a result of a squint in childhood. Not taking an appropriate visual history can result in unnecessary referrals to ophthalmology clinics.

VA is best measured using the 6m method (a patient sitting 6m from the Snellen chart), which may be set up using mirrors in small rooms, for example, with two 3m distances. Adapted Snellen charts are also available with the same apparent letter size to the person at shorter distances of 3m.

Normal VA is around the 6/6 (6/4 to 6/9) level, but may vary particularly with lighting level, refractive error, amblyopia, and variable glucose control (see Chapter 4).

To measure VA:

- Position the patient directly facing the VA chart
- Start with the right eye, first occluding the fellow eye
- If glasses or lenses are worn for distance vision, ensure the patient is wearing them
- Record how vision was measured, that is, unaided/with glasses or with pinhole.
  VA is measured by distance and size of letters, that is, 6/12:
- Top figure 6 = distance in metres between patient and chart
- Bottom figure 12 = the last complete line the patient reads

If the patient is unable to read the top line at 6m (6/60), take them to a 3m distance and measure as before. This alters the readings to 3/60.

If the patient is still unable to read top letter at 3m then

- A recording of C/F (count fingers) is made by holding two or three fingers at a distance of 1m or
- A recording of hand movements (HM) by holding your hand about 1m away and gently waving the hand
- The next level is perception of light (PL) or no perception of light (NPL)
- Repeat VA recording for the other eye.

10.3 **Drop instillation using mydriasis**

Check that VA has already been tested and recorded.
Patients must be warned prior to a screening visit by letter:

- NOT TO DRIVE for 2–5 hours afterwards. This should be clearly stipulated in patient information leaflets or invite letters
- ALWAYS check allergy status before instilling any drops into the eyes; if unsure seek advice
- Ensure correct patient identification (ask the patient for their date of birth, address, or other identifiers if unsure)
- Ensure local infection control hand-washing procedure is followed
- Topical tropicamide 1% solution at one drop is the common dilating agent used. Apply drops to the fornix which ensures that the agent is maximally absorbed
- The iris usually needs a minimum of 20 minutes for adequate pupil dilation before commencing retinal photography
- If there is insufficient pupil dilatation with one drop of 1% tropicamide as described above, a repeat of tropicamide in addition to phenylephrine 2.5% should be instilled (Birmingham protocol).

10.4 **Contraindications to pupil dilation**

10.4.1 **Dilating patients with glaucoma?**

The concern and contraindication of pharmacological pupil dilation in patients with glaucoma has become embedded in medicine. The concern arises from the risk of precipitation of acute glaucoma in patients with narrow anterior chamber angle. This is a very rare event, and does not occur in patients with known glaucoma as appropriate treatment (e.g. iridotomy for closed angle glaucoma) will have been performed, thereby making pupil dilation safe. The common open-angle glaucoma can be dilated safely. However, patients should be warned in patient information leaflets that if someone develops the suggestive symptoms of acute glaucoma including acute pain and a red eye hours after mydriasis, they should report urgently to a hospital eye casualty department.

10.4.2 **Iris clip lens**

Up to 1984, an intra-ocular lens implant used following cataract extraction was an iris clip lens, placed in the anterior chamber of the eye (see Figure 10.3). This lens was held in place by studs on the pupil surface, such that pupil dilation would result in anterior dislocation of the prosthetic lens. This resulted in a disgruntled patient because of visual distortion and the requirement for further ocular surgery. The presence of this type of lens can be detected by anterior chamber photography as in Figure 10.3, and is an absolute contraindication to mydriasis.

10.4.3 **Patient Group Directive (PGD)**

As of 2007, in the United Kingdom, it has been an essential advance to allow retinal screeners to perform VA and mydriasis without medical supervision. Most hospitals and screening programmes will have protocols for a PGD agreement to instill mydriatic drops without a doctor's signed prescription each time—it may be a pre-printed prescription allowing staff to check VA and to instill dilating drops using a standard protocol, stressing safe practice with appropriate exclusions and advice about not driving following mydriasis.

Figure 10.3 An iris clip lens

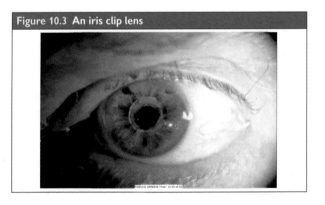

10.5 Taking acceptable digital retinal images

A retinal screener's role is to obtain the best possible images, thus gathering and recording correct information from the photography session. It is imperative to ascertain whether the patient is already under diabetic eye clinic care, as screening is therefore inappropriate appropriate (i.e. the patients by definition have referable disease).

The photographic process is:

- Position the patient comfortably. Ask the patient to rest their chin on the rest and forehead, correctly aligning the patient's eyes with the camera alignment markers (see Figure 10.4)
- Explain what they will experience, for example: a bright flash. Ask the patient to follow the green internal or external fixation light (some fixators being external).
- Move camera sliding base forwards, returning the camera mirror control (a button on the top of the sliding camera base) until the retina is clearly visible. Adjust the focusing control and joystick until the correct field is obtained
- Take an optic disc and a macula-centred view for each eye respectively (see Figure 10.5). This is standard for the English screening programme, but there are variations in other programmes, for example, using a single macula view only
- Other settings will be needed for illumination and camera flash which will be specified by camera manufacturers.

Figure 10.4 Eye alignment with the camera lens

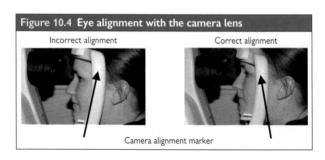

Incorrect alignment · Correct alignment

Camera alignment marker

10.5.1 **Anterior chamber (AC) photography**

If the retinal view is hazy, our policy is to photograph an anterior chamber view. To do this,

- Keep the camera compensation filters (magnification lens dioptres to adjust for + or − normal refractive changes) pull control fully out
- Adjust so that the front of the eye (anterior chamber) is showing on the camera monitor
- Focus on the pupil (set to fine focus, thus sharpening the image)
- Take the photograph.

Examples of the value of anterior chamber photographs are shown in Chapters 4, 8 and 10 (Figures 4.1, 4.5, 8.8 and 10.3), for example, demonstrating the different types of cataracts and other abnormalities.

Figure 10.5 The two standard views obtained, one centred on the macula and the other on the optic disc

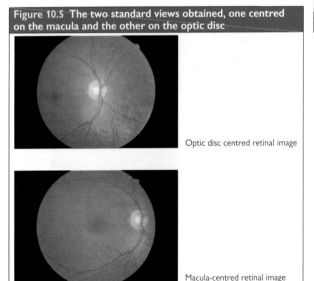

Optic disc centred retinal image

Macula-centred retinal image

10.6 **Problems with digital fundal photography**

Camera operational problems you CAN control

- Dark photos (Figure 10.6)—Often due to poor pupil dilation; increase the flash level or leave for longer dilation. May need more mydriatics
- Rim artefact (Figure 10.7)—Check patient's head is resting on chin rest facing squarely straight ahead
- Circle photographic artefact (Figure 10.8)—Pull the camera out and re-position if the camera alignment is incorrect (the camera may be too close, too far away, or not over the centre of the retina).

Figure 10.6 Dark photos

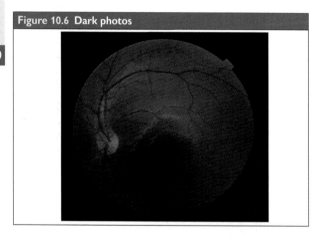

Problems you CAN'T control

- Cataract may result in an ungradable digital image (Figure 11.3) and may have to be referred into ophthalmology for slit lamp bio-microscopy examination
- Asteroides hyalosis are particles in the vitreous due to calcium soaps and commonly result in ungradable photographs (see Figures 9.18 and 10.9). It may be difficult to distinguish whether the opacities in the vitreous are asteroides particles or exudates as they can look identical in appearance. Patients may need to have retinal screening performed long term by slit lamp bio-microscopy examination in the hospital eye service

- Artefacts on the camera lens—marks on the camera lens may cause artefacts which may compromise the fundal image area, making the image difficult to grade or mistaken for retinal pathology (see Figure 10.10). Other small dots and black artefacts may appear on an image, which are caused by dust settling on the camera chip due to static build up. This should result in obtaining specialist help from the camera suppliers.

Figure 10.7 'Rim artefact'

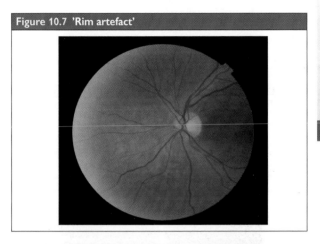

Figure 10.8 The 'circle artefact'

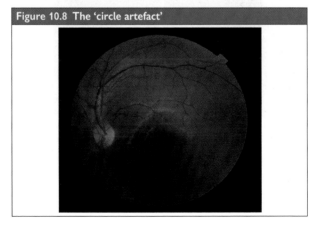

Figure 10.9 Asteroides hyalosis

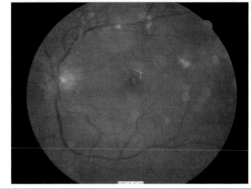

Figure 10.10 This is a lens artefact as it occupies the same position in the photograph regardless of centration and/or the eye

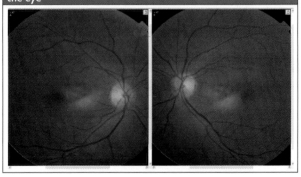

10.7 **NSC standards/targets of acceptable image quality**

- 2 × nominal 45° fields per eye (see Figure 10.5)
- A macula-centred view field is taken so that any maculopathy can be clearly detected and a disc (nasal) view can assist detecting pre-proliferative retinopathy in the periphery of the retina (R2) and proliferative retinopathy (R3)
- Taking two views helps with detecting artefacts or reflection which disappear or move on one of the two views taken
- Images are only to be utilized if the grader is confident with the quality of the screening photographs (see section 11.4).

Chapter 11

How to grade

Helen C King

> **Key points**
> - The grading environment should be quiet, with appropriate lighting, and grading undertaken on high-quality computer equipment and screens.
> - A grader needs good pattern recognition skills and attention to detail.
> - Graders should adhere to minimum standards and numbers of grades as required by the NSC.
> - A grading scheme has been formulated comprising a retinopathy grade (R) and a maculopathy grade (M).
> - Graders should check image quality, and use a step-by-step grading method which may also use image manipulation.

11.1 The grading environment

The environment that a grader works in is very important to ensure that grading is consistently accurate. The equipment that a grader requires cannot be compromised and the room should be adequately darkened, preventing any glare on the computer screen which may interfere with their view of images. The room should be as quiet as possible, with distractions kept to a minimum, helping to maximize concentration. Where possible, graders should be working in close proximity to other competent graders who can give advice—helping to increase a grader's confidence and allowing a team to learn from one another. A grading laboratory is such an environment used in the Birmingham scheme, (Figure 11.1).

11.2 The job profile of a grader

Graders can come from any background, as long as they have the key skills required for all graders:
- Good pattern recognition
- Fast learning skills
- Attention to detail
- Adequate training to be competent to grade.

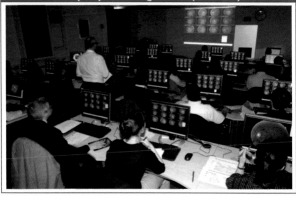

Figure 11.1 The grading laboratory of the Heart of England Diabetic Retinopathy Screening Centre (HEDRSC)

An optimum workload for a grader, along with the necessary training and maintenance of expertise, is essential to maintain skills, grading accuracy, and job satisfaction. Recommendations from the National Screening Committee (NSC) is that graders should have a 10-minute break after every solid hour of grading, and should spend no longer than half a day grading at a time. More than this does prove tiring, thereby increasing the risk of human error and therefore leading to incorrect grading.

One of the key objectives of a screening scheme is to have high sensitivity and specificity, thereby preventing false positives (unnecessary referrals) and false negatives (non-referral of referable images). The accuracy of grading is key to this and will make the difference between a screening scheme being successful or not.

There are also NSC Guidelines for optometrists which state that they should grade a minimum of 500 patients' image sets per annum to participate as a grader within a screening scheme in England. Graders, other than optometrists should grade a minimum of 1000 patients' image sets per annum to maintain their expertise. Tertiary graders (usually senior ophthalmologist) should grade more than 500 patient image sets per annum for their accreditation.

11.2.1 **Non-grading photographers**

There are no guidelines from the NSC for non-grading photographers, who may simply capture the retinal images; However, it is mandatory that they have appropriate training and supervised, thereby taking excellent, relevant images and accelerate image grading where necessary. It is also important that a relevant visual history is taken if the visual acuity is abnormal, and training in this element is essential.

11.3 **How to grade?**

11.3.1 **The National Grading Minimum Dataset**

The local grading standards for all retinopathy screening programmes within England should include the English Retinopathy Minimum Grading Standards devised by the NSC. This is because of the need to compare different results from the grading of different populations and screening programmes nationwide, and also to facilitate national audit.

Small local variations may apply at the discretion of the clinical lead, but are additional, in grades or subdivisions of the national grading criteria.

The national grading minimum dataset: Each eye photographed should receive a retinopathy 'R grade' and a maculopathy 'M grade'.

11.3.2 **Retinopathy grading: 'The R grade'**

The R grade indicates the level of retinopathy for the retinal views in question (i.e. using both images).

- *R0* (None): No visible diabetic retinopathy (DR)
- *R1* (Background DR): Microaneurysm(s) and/or retinal haemorrhages with or without exudates anywhere on the retina (see Chapter 5)
- *R2* (Pre-proliferative DR): Venous beading, venous looping, re-duplication, intra-retinal microvascular abnormalities (IRMAs), multiple deep, round, or blot haemorrhages, many cotton wool spots along with other features above (see Chapter 7)
- *R3* (Proliferative DR): New vessels elsewhere (NVE), new vessels on the disc (NVD) (see Chapter 7), pre-retinal haemorrhage/vitreous haemorrhage, pre-retinal fibrosis with or without tractional retinal detachment (see Chapters 7 and 8).

11.3.3 **Maculopathy grading 'The M grade'**

The M grade indicates the amount of diabetic retinopathy within the critical macula region (see Chapter 6) of the eye (maculopathy):

M0 (No maculopathy) No exudates within the macula region, or haemorrhages and/or microaneurysm(s) within the macula region with VA 6/9 and better

M1 (Referable maculopathy) An eye should be graded as M1 if there is

• Exudate within 1 disc diameter (DD) of the centre of the fovea; see (Chapter 6, Figure 6.5)

OR

• A circinate (circle of exudates) or a group of exudates within the macula (2DD of the centre of the fovea) (Chapter 6, Figure 6.6)

OR

• Any microaneurysm and/or haemorrhage within 1DD of the centre of the fovea if accompanied by a VA of 6/12 or worse.

If there is any maculopathy present then the R grade must be a minimum of R1 (as this means that there is a minimum of background retinopathy on the whole retina).

11.3.4 **Patient outcomes from grading**

Table 11.1	
DR Grade	**Outcome**
R0M0 No DR Present	ANNUAL RECALL
R1M0 (Background, no maculopathy)	ANNUAL RECALL
R2M0 (Pre-proliferative + no maculopathy)	ROUTINE REFERRAL TO HES*
R1M1 (Maculopathy)	ROUTINE REFERRAL TO HES
R2M1 (Pre-proliferative and maculopathy)	ROUTINE REFERRAL TO HES
R3M0 (Proliferative + no maculopathy)	URGENT REFERRAL TO HES
R3M1 (Proliferative + maculopathy)	URGENT REFERRAL TO HES
U (Ungradable image)	ROUTINE REFERRAL TO HES
Other Lesions	REFERRED AS OF LOCAL PROTOCOLS
* HES = Hospital eye service.	

11.3.5 **Other gradings**

Presence of laser

If a retina has had previous laser treatment (see Chapter 7, Figure 7.7, Figure 11.5 and Chapter 17), then the laser treatment type should be assessed. This will either have been for treatment of new vessels or for maculopathy.

Where laser is present, the retina should be graded using the standard gradings with the addition of 'P' for photocoagulation. This will be included in the screening software.

11.4 **Image quality**

As described in Chapter 10, two 45° fields of each eye should be captured, a foveal-centred and a disc-centred view, the grading should take into account both of these views, together with an assessment of both the position and image quality (clarity) of each field. The quality of an image can be classed as good, adequate, or inadequate (i.e. ungradable). See classifications provided in the following sections (Figure 11.2).

11.4.1 **Good view-macular centred image**

Position: The centre of the fovea should be within, or 1DD from the centre of the image.

Clarity: Vessels should be clearly visible within 1DD of the centre of the fovea.

11.4.2 **Good view-disc centred image**

Position: The centre of the disc should be within 1DD of the centre of the image.

Clarity: Vessels should be clearly visible on the surface of the disc.

For images to be classed as 'Good' vessels should be visible across 90% of the image.

11.4.3 **Adequate view-macular centred image**

Position: The centre of the fovea should be over 2DD from the edge of the image, ensuring that the 45° view can be seen, with nothing being missed off the edge of the retina.

11.4.4 **Adequate view-disc centred image**

Position: The whole optic disc should be over 2DD from the edge of the image, with the fine vessels visible on the surface of the disc.

Failure to meet the standards of an adequate view mean that images should be graded as ungradable (U) and referred as routine unless urgent referable retinopathy is visible anywhere on the image (i.e. *de novo* R3).

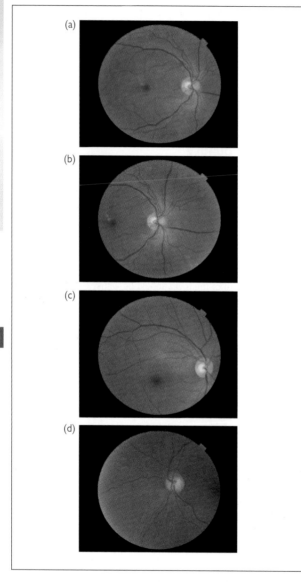

Figure 11.2 (a) A macular view classed as 'Good'. (b) A disc view classed as 'Good'. (c) A macular view classed as 'adequate'. (d) A disc view classed as 'adequate'.

There should be local bio-microscopy clinics set up to screen patients who are unassessable by digital photography. Only accredited and competent staff should be performing grading, at various levels. If a grader is not confident because of the quality of an image, regardless of the standards set earlier they should refer the images as unassessable to allow a senior member of staff to decide the outcome.

The percentage of ungradable images will vary from scheme to scheme depending on the incidence of untreated cataract. The national minimum standard is that there should be no more than 10% ungradable images in a screening scheme.

11.5 **Image manipulation**

Using digital photography to screen patients allows us a host of image manipulation tools to enhance the quality of the images, graders should try their best to grade an image using these tools before referring it as unassessable (Figure 11.3).

However, brightening up and over manipulation of an image can cause an image to become grainy and more difficult to grade. Manipulation also takes up time and so should be used only on images where it is necessary. Similarly, altering the contrast of an image can be useful, but too much of this can lead to a pixelated image, and make diabetic retinopathy more difficult to detect.

Using red-free manipulation can be useful as it shows up and contrasts vascular abnormalities more clearly. It is a useful technique for identifying microaneurysms and exudates, but particularly useful in the diagnosis of new vessels on an image, which may be difficult to see on a colour image (see Figures 11.4 and 11.5).

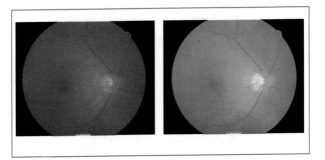

Figure 11.3 The left image shows a hazy dark view due to cataract and poor dilatation, the right image shows the same image brightened up using enhancement software making the maculopathy much clearer to see.

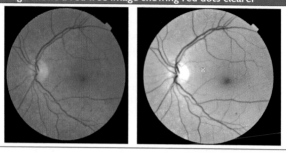

Figure 11.4 The left image shows a colour image and the right image shows a red-free image showing red dots clearer

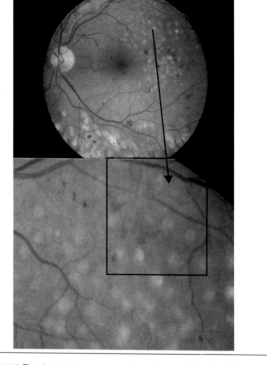

Figure 11.5 This shows in the top pane a colour photograph showing old laser treatment, but no obvious new vessels. The red-free enhanced view in the lower panel demonstrates that there are clearly NVE in the superior temporal region (highlighted in the square box).

11.6 **Step-by-step guide to grading**

Every grader will have their own method for grading; here is a step-by-step guide to ensuring that every part of the retina is checked and graded sufficiently.

1. Check VA
   - This may affect the grade/outcome?
   - Do you require more information/history from patient?
2. Enlarge macula-centred (right or left) view
   - What is the image quality—is the image assessable?
3. Magnify the macula and assess for M grade (maculopathy)
   - Either MO or M1.
4. Look at the rest of the retina and vasculature on the macular view and assess for R grade (retinopathy) or any other lesions
   - Either R0, R1, R2, or R3.
5. Enlarge the optic disc view and assess for quality.
6. Magnify the optic disc and assess for any DR or other lesions.
7. Look at the rest of the retina on the optic disc view and assess for R (retinopathy) grade or any other lesions, and confirm the M grade.
8. Enlarge any previous images
   - Compare any abnormalities/assess changes, and read comments.
9. Input the grade ± comments into the software, and do the same with the other eye.

Whilst this schemata is only a rough guide used by our graders, it is clear that lesions will be missed if a system is not employed by each individual and appropriate time is not spent on each set of images. Grading timings and accuracy do also reflect practice and experience with pattern recognition, such that graders do need supervision and support in the initial months until all are confident in grading accuracy.

113

Further reading

National Screening Committee Service Objectives and Quality Assurance Standards (6) (2007).

National Screening Committee. UK National Screening Committee Workbook 4 (August 2007); 77–8.

Scanlon PH, Malhotra R, Thomas G, Foy C, Kirkpatrick JN, Lewis-Barned N, et al. The effectiveness of screening for diabetic retinopathy by digital imaging photography and technician ophthalmoscopy. Diabetic Medicine 2003; **20**(6): 467–74.

Chapter 12

The principles of a national diabetic retinopathy screening programme

Margaret Clarke

Key Points

A The *aim of the programme* is to reduce the risk of sight loss among people with diabetes by the prompt identification and effective treatment of sight-threatening retinopathy at the appropriate stage during the disease process.

B A diabetic retinopathy screening programme consists of several key components:
1. Administration in place
2. Digital retinal cameras available
3. Trained and accredited screening/grading staff
4. Grading pathways—to include quality assurance
5. Quality assurance—both internal and external
6. Appropriate referrals to ophthalmologist
7. Laser treatment and referrals seen in a timely manner
8. Information systems to manage and report all of the above
9. Comprehensive annual reports.

12.1 Introduction

The policy for screening for diabetic retinopathy (DR) has been clearly set out in the National Service Framework for Diabetes. A work book is available which lays out all the details required for the English screening programme, and covers all aspects in some detail. This is available online (www.retinalscreening.co.uk). The other three nations in the UK have similar statements which contain variations, but are in broad agreement. Although a National Programme local policy is being implemented by individual programmes, a number of key factors have been recommended. The principles of these will now be outlined.

12.2 **Who to screen?**

All persons with diabetes aged 12yrs and above should be offered screening for sight-threatening DR using digital retinal photography. It is not thought necessary to screen those already under the care of diabetic eye clinics.

12.3 **Screening programme size and administration**

It is stated that all screening programmes should cover at least 12 000 people with diabetes (ie serving a general population of approximately 500 000). Programmes need to be sufficiently large to enable meaningful data to be collected and to ensure enough exposure of images to enable expertise amongst graders.

The administration needs to achieve the following:

- A single collated list of all people with diabetes in the community, that is, a register and mechanisms for adding and removing diabetic subjects
- Organization of screening appointments including follow up of non-attenders
- Linkage with ophthalmic services for those already under the care of an ophthalmologist
- Formal annual audit of screening uptake and coverage
- Quality assurance system in place
- System of recall of screen-positive patients.

12.4 **Screening programme models**

There are four main models of screening programmes which have been adopted, but there are a number of combinations of models being used:

- Fixed location screening services where the service is supplied through one or more static units, such as cameras in a hospital or diabetes centre
- Mobile screening services where the service is provided at a range of locations, such as GP surgeries or from a mobile screening van
- Optometry-based services where the central administration of the programme directs patients to accredited optometrists
- Mixed services which may involve any or all of the above or other external agencies.

The majority of schemes are based on mobile cameras (see Figure 12.1), but a number of them are based on community screening by optometrists with digital cameras in their practices. Providing there are 12 000 diabetes patients and a central call/recall system and central administration, then where the delivery takes place will be determined at a local level. A central grading facility is also important.

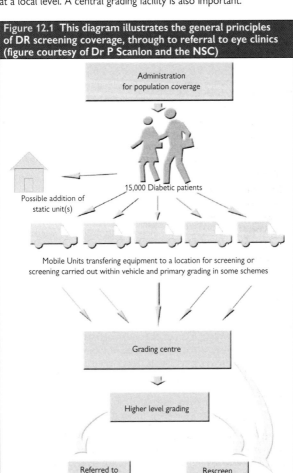

Figure 12.1 This diagram illustrates the general principles of DR screening coverage, through to referral to eye clinics (figure courtesy of Dr P Scanlon and the NSC)

Administration for population coverage

15,000 Diabetic patients

Possible addition of static unit(s)

Mobile Units transfering equipment to a location for screening or screening carried out within vehicle and primary grading in some schemes

Grading centre

Higher level grading

Referred to ophthalmology

Rescreen 1 year

12.5 **The screening appointment**

Care should be taken to ensure that the identity of the person being screened is securely established by

- Asking to see the letter of appointment and double checking the NHS number against the patient record
- Asking the individual to state his or her full name, address, and date of birth
- Check that the details match the patient record.

The screening appointment should include two digital colour photographs of each eye after mydriasis by a trained and accredited screener, as in Chapter 10.

12.5.1 **Communication of results**

Results should be communicated to **all** patients in writing as soon as possible, as well as to the clinicians providing their diabetic care. The concept of 'no news is good news' is not acceptable in a national screening programme. The standard is that the result should be available and posted within 3 weeks of the screening episode.

12.5.2 **What can the screener tell the patient?**

The time that the photograph is taken may be a good opportunity for patient education on the importance of screening, and the significance of the result. However, these results have not been quality assured, graded, and therefore may not be the definitive result.

Whilst it is desirable for patients to be shown the images if they wish to view them and for general information to be given about the retina and diabetic retinopathy, great care must be taken not to mislead the patient about the outcome of the grading process. They should be told that a careful scrutiny of the images using appropriate equipment will be undertaken and checked, and that the final result will be given in writing. It is our policy that patients who need urgent referral will however need to be advised of this, to ensure that they can make themselves available at short notice for an eye clinic appointment.

The decision as to whether screeners and graders will give verbal interim feedback has been designated as the responsibility of the clinical lead for each programme in the English scheme.

12.5.3 **Roles within the screening programme: definitions**

- *Screener*—describes anyone involved in the process of identification of sight-threatening diabetic retinopathy in a screening programme for diabetic retinopathy (including grading). This group may include medical photographers, healthcare assistants, GPs, diabetologists, ophthalmologists, and optometrists.

- *Grader*—examines the retinal images for evidence of diabetic change in the eye and assesses those images for disease against the minimum dataset. Primary graders assess for first grade, while secondary graders assess all abnormal and 10% of normal grades.
- *Arbitration grader*—carries out grading in the event that there is disagreement between the primary and secondary grader. Usually this will be done by an ophthalmologist or an experienced screener, accredited to the highest level.
- *Tertiary grader*— is an experienced senior clinician, usually an ophthalmologist or an appropriately skilled diabetologist, who decides on clinical outcome, that is, whether referral to the hospital eye services is needed.

12.6 **Grading pathways**

Any grading should include the English Retinopathy Minimum Grading Classifications as discussed in Chapters 4–8, and 11. The National Screening Programme has been developed primarily to detect sight-threatening diabetic retinopathy and not to detect other eye conditions. However, other eye conditions may be detected during routine grading, and local protocols need to be in place for their management (see Chapter 9).

The recommendation is that all graders grade a minimum of 1000 image sets each year. The type of grade should be appropriate to their level of accreditation. A description of the principles of the grading pathway outlined by the English DR screening programme are shown in Figures 12.2 and 12.3. This outlines small variations according to initial grader skills, but the more common full-grader pathway is illustrated in Figure 12.3 and is:

- *Stage 1*: A grader accredited to do so carries out a full disease grading on all image sets. Urgent referrals (R3) should be passed to the grading centre for immediate assessment by an ophthalmologist.
- *Stage 2*: A different grader will assess a random 10% of the no disease image sets and carry out a second full grading on all the disease image sets from the stage 1 grade. That second grader should not see the result of the first grader prior to grading.
- *Arbitration*: If there is a difference of opinion between the two full disease graders, then those image sets should be referred onwards for an arbitration grade by a suitably qualified and experienced professional who will decide whether the patient should be referred to the ophthalmology service or back into the screening programme.

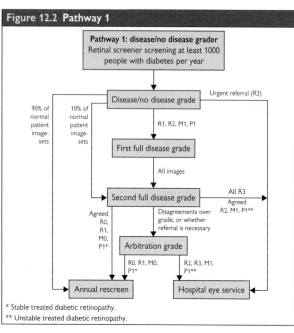

Figure 12.2 Pathway 1

* Stable treated diabetic retinopathy.
** Unstable treated diabetic retinopathy.

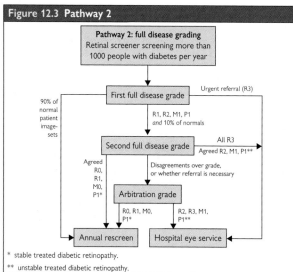

Figure 12.3 Pathway 2

* stable treated diabetic retinopathy.
** unstable treated diabetic retinopathy.

Sets of images with referable retinopathy, ungradable images, or other lesions should be referred for tertiary grading by an experienced senior clinician, usually an ophthalmologist or an appropriately skilled diabetologist.

12.7 Quality assurance (QA)

There are two categories of QA:

- Internal QA forms part of the every day processes in a screening programme.
- External quality assurance is a completely objective assessment of programmes and there is a comparative analysis of the outcomes.

Both are essential aspects of any screening programme. The purpose of QA is to

- Reduce the probability of error
- Ensure that errors are dealt with competently and sensitively
- Help professionals and organizations improve year on year
- Set and re-set standards (national responsibility).

Specific standards have been set for screening programmes, at two levels—a minimum and achievable level—and a summary of these are outlined as an Appendix to this chapter.

In essence the internal QA to be performed is
10% of all normals are regraded and checked (R0M0)
and
All abnormal sets of images (R1 and/or M1 or greater).

All screening programmes should close the loop with an audit of screening failures, to review the screening history, and previous images/results where appropriate.

It is necessary to monitor both disease negatives, to ensure that disease is not being missed, and disease positives, to minimize inappropriate referrals (and associated patient anxiety).

All disease-positive cases should be reviewed prior to issue of a referral appointment—this will also ensure prompt referral of serious disease to an ophthalmology clinic without overloading clinics and causing unnecessary alarm to patients. The screening and grading pathway needs to be followed closely to ensure that clinically significant data are accurately assessed and referred promptly where appropriate. In the Birmingham scheme, approximately 40–50% of patient image sets are being quality assurance regraded.

Programmes should measure their performance against the national quality standards, and complete an annual report on their year-end performance. The primary purpose of the report is to enable effective self-review and to provide a structured method against which to assess the strengths and weaknesses of programmes against the set standards.

Summary

The main essentials of a systematic DR screening programme are described, from screening through to the grading and referral process. It is an ambitious project to put in place, but is already bearing rewards, with trained accredited staff, reports being made, patients attending screening, and above all, delivering the target of reduction in visual loss in our diabetic patients.

Appendix—Standards to be achieved

The NSC has listed 19 standards that should be achieved by screening programmes in England. They set minimum and achievable levels. The principles with their objectives and minimum and achievable standards (www.retinalscreening.co.uk) are now outlined:

Standard 1. Objective—to reduce new blindness due to diabetic retinopathy

- To be measured by collecting annual blind and partially sighted registration rates predominantly due to diabetes and compared to 1990/1991 rates of 9.5 and 9.3, respectively per million per year (national data).
- Minimum standard: 10% reduction within 5 years.
- Achievable standard: 40% reduction within 5 years.

Standard 2. Objective—to identify and invite all eligible persons with known diabetes to attend for the DR screening test

- To ensure the maximum number of persons are screened and recalled as appropriate.
- Proportion of GPs participating (minimum standard 90%, achievable standard 98%).
- Proportion of known people with diabetes on register (minimum standard 90%, achievable standard 98%).
- Single collated list of all people with diabetes.
- Systematic call/recall from a single centre of all people eligible for screening on the collated list.

Standard 3. Objective—to ensure database is accurate

• To ensure that letters, results, etc., are sent to appropriate individuals
• The accuracy of addresses on database of persons aged 12 or more, will be assessed by Post Office returns (minimum standard 95%, achievable standard 98%).

Standard 4. Objective—to maximize the number of invited persons accepting the test

Minimum standard:

1. Initial screen—70% eligible persons accepting the test
2. Repeat screen—80% eligible persons accepting the test.

Achievable standard:

1. Initial screen—90% eligible persons accepting the test
2. Repeat screen—95% eligible persons accepting the test.

Standard 5. Objective—to ensure photographs are of adequate quality

Inadequate photographs cause increased cost and inconvenience.

This will be measured by recording the percentage ungradable patients in at least one eye, including cataracts (minimum standard <10%; achievable standard <5%), and percentage ungradable patients in at least one eye, once cataracts have been excluded (minimum standard <5%; achievable standard <3%).

Standard 6. Objective—to ensure grading is accurate

Assess inter- and intra-grader agreement for referable, non referable and ungradable images.

Standard 7 for Optometrists —Objective—to ensure optimum workload for graders and to maintain expertise

Minimum standard: Each optometrist should grade a minimum of 500 image sets each year.

Achievable standard: Each grader should grade a minimum of 1500 patient image sets per annum.

Regular breaks should be taken whilst grading to guard against errors due to fatigue.

Standard 8. Objective —to ensure timely referral of abnormal screening results (e-mailed or posted)

Time between screen and grading when flagged by screener as fast-track referral (i.e. urgent).

Minimum standard:
95% referred within 1 calendar week
100% referred within 2 calendar weeks.

Achievable standard:
98% referred within 1 week.

Standard 9. Objective —to ensure that both GP and patient are informed of all test results

Time before posting notification letters to GP and patient.

Minimum standard:

70% in less than 3 weeks
100% in less than 6 weeks.

Achievable standard:

95% in less than 3 weeks.

Standard 10. Objective—to ensure timely consultation for all screen-positive patients

Minimum standard:

   Time between notification of positive test and consultation:

   1. Proliferative DR (R3)—70% in less than 2 weeks
   2. Pre-proliferative DR, R2—70% in less than 13 weeks
   3. Maculopathy, M1—70% in less than 13 weeks
   4. All retinopathy grades—less than 18 weeks.

Standard 11. Objective—to ensure timely treatment of those listed by ophthalmologist

Minimum standard:

   Time between listing and first laser:

   1. Proliferative DR—90% in less than 2 weeks
   2. Maculopathy—70% in less than 10 weeks.

Standard 12. Objective—to minimize overall delay between screening event and first laser

Minimum standard:

   Time between screening and first laser does not exceed

   1. For patients referred as R3—70% within 4 weeks.
   2. 100% in less than 6 weeks
   3. For patients referred as M1—70% within 15 weeks.
   4. 100% in less than 26 weeks.

Standard 13. Objective—to follow up screen-positive patients.

Minimum standard:

   DNA rate for ophthalmology clinic:

   1. For PDR (R3) within 1 month, less than 10%
   2. For PPDR (R2) within 6 months, less than 10%
   3. Maculopathy within 6 months, less than 10%.

Standard 14. Objective—to minimize the anxiety associated with screening

Measure:

   Monitor inappropriate referrals following screening:

   1. False positive rate of DR test (photograph)

2. Neither photograph or clinical examination warranted referral.
Minimum standard: <25% of patients referred.

Standard 15. Objective—to ensure timely rescreening
To ensure there is a truly annual screening and patients are not left for too long (risking disease progression), or screened too soon (causing increased cost).

Minimum standard: 70% of patients re-screened within 12 months of the previous screening encounter or 95% re-screened within 15 months of the previous screening encounter.

Standard 16. Objective—to ensure that the public and health care professionals are informed at regular intervals
Measure and standard: Timely production of annual report.

Standard 17. Objective—to ensure that the scheme participates in quality assurance
This will be assessed by external quality assurance.

Standard 18. Objective—to optimize programme efficiency and ensure ability to assure quality of service
Minimum programme size of 12 000 people diagnosed with diabetes on the current patient list.

Achievable standard: 15 000 people diagnosed with diabetes on the current patient list.

Standard 19. Objective—to ensure that all screening and grading of retinal images are provided by a trained and accredited workforce
All staff must be accredited for their role within 2 years of appointment.

Chapter 13

Programme administration

Helen C King and Caroline Harrison

Key points

A systematic screening programme should have
- An accurate patient register
- Central call/recall for subjects
- Tight, monitored, and auditable exclusion criteria for subjects
- The capacity to produce annual reports
- Well-organized administrative service.

13.1 Introduction

Effective administration is essential to ensure a consistent approach to a screening programme so that it functions effectively, is monitored, and there is maintenance of quality and safety measures. A clear structure needs to be in place identifying roles and responsibilities with procedures in place for all those involved in the administration of the scheme. The pathway through the scheme does involve communication, and contact with several healthcare professionals and organizations which needs co-coordination. The administration of the scheme also needs to have all the necessary protocols in place. This will include clinical and information governance, adherence to data protection and security, sharing protocols in place where required between organizations, and password and security protocols for data protection.

13.2 Patient list for diabetic retinopathy (DR) screening

For each screening scheme there should be a single collated list of patients confirmed to have diabetes who are over the age of 12. The data required for each of these patients is full name, date of birth, NHS number, and general practitioners' (GPs) names and contact details.

To collect and maintain this list a consistent exchange of data with GP practices is essential. As the prevalence of diabetes is increasing, this list will grow and confirmed patient's details will change, some may change address and GP, and some decease.

It is imperative that the screening database has

- Frequent updates and management
- Good links with GP practices is essential to ensure the register remains accurate
- Good data quality controls in place
- System maintenance reports
- Secure electronic links between the scheme and GP practices, so that data can be exchanged securely and acted on in a timely manner
- Exchange of information for newly diagnosed diabetics, changes to patient's details (change of address, moved out of the area, and deceased).

There needs to be investment in time for the GP registers of diabetic patients to be recorded on a centralized system, so that GP practices can check with their practice register their accuracy on a regular basis and report any changes and additions. This helps build good relationships with general practitioners by keeping them informed of developments, changes to the service, and identifying issues such as low uptake of screening, that is, being proactive. Schemes that have operated separate lists, based within separate GP/optometry practices have had problems when required to collate data and synchronize invitations and appointments, which can lead to many patients not being identified. The English diabetic retinopathy (DR) screening programme, therefore, suggests a single comprehensive list and a single call/recall centre to most effective.

The patient list should be separated into subgroups (Figure 13.1).

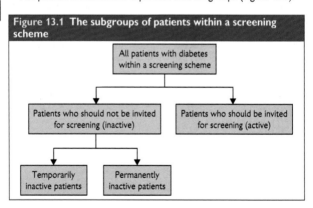

Figure 13.1 The subgroups of patients within a screening scheme

The active list of patients with diabetes is those who should receive invitations to screening appointments annually.

Temporarily inactive: Patients put on the temporary inactive list should not receive invitations to screening for a certain period of time. This amount of time should either be decided by the patient or by a healthcare professional, usually the GP or ophthalmologist, allowing the patient to re-participate fully after the amount of time. Screening software systems will usually allow you to set the date and automatically send an invitation out after the period of time.

Permanently inactive: Patients put on the permanently inactive list will not be invited for screening unless they are moved to the temporarily inactive list or the active list, that is, they are excluded from the screening programme.

Call/recall: Having one centralized managed call/recall system is a major advantage for the following:

• Monitoring and organizing the whole cohort of patients
• Reducing the amount of complex communication between different call/recall centres
• Allowing systematic coverage of the entire geographical area
• Sending invitations to be spread out across the year
• Giving the ability to plan for the workload within the administration and screening/grading capacity
• Letters and patient information that is standardized across a scheme, making it streamlined, recognizable
• Reducing confusion for patients.

Without a central call/recall system a large amount of extra workload is generated. It may delay result letters and have an impact on the quality of work. It may also have an impact on eye departments, increasing workload and waiting list times. A single, collated list of patients within each programme may be inaccurate, leading to risk of safety and effectiveness of the whole programme because patients will be missed. The timeliness of the whole administration process is paramount to the success of the programme. The whole process needs to be systematic and fully managed.

The *Standards* that are set for the English programme relating to administration are numbers 2, 3, 4, and 15 as outlined in the Appendix of Chapter 12.

13.2 **Annual reporting for DR screening programmes**

Reporting is a key administrative function. Reports are needed to identify

- Data quality
- Timeliness of the recording of patient information
- Identification of trends or patterns in activity that may need investigation
- Comparison of data on a national basis, for example, effectiveness, trends, prevalence of DR, treatment and visual outcomes, and how a scheme is performing against national standards compared to others.

The annual report recommended by the NSC is vital to this and can be compared year on year, which should identify strengths and weaknesses of the programme. This enables review of all aspects and to identify areas that can be targeted where improvements are needed.

13.3 **Exclusions from DR screening**

Every screening scheme will have a small number of their diabetic population who are not eligible for screening. It is essential that the scheme audits those patients who have been excluded on an annual basis to check that they have been excluded for valid reasons. GPs have an important role to play as well by ensuring that patients who are to be excluded have received sufficient information to make this choice.

The principles for patient exclusion are as follows:

Patient choice: A small number of patients who are eligible for screening will not want to be part of the screening programme. If a patient has decided to opt out, it is very important that they have been given all of the necessary information for this to be an informed choice for that patient. If the patient still wants to be excluded, then they should be encouraged to join the temporarily inactive list, so that they can be re-invited.

The individual should confirm their decision in writing, sending the letter to their GP and to the screening scheme.

Under the age of 12: Patients with diabetes are not eligible for screening until they are 12 years old.

13.3.1 Consent for screening

Children aged 16 and above are deemed competent to give informed consent to be screened.

Children below age 16 are deemed as competent to give informed consent to be screened if the child has 'sufficient understanding and intelligence to enable him or her to fully understand what is proposed'.

In cases where the child is not competent to give an informed decision the person with parental responsibility must give their consent for the child to be screened. It is, however, encouraged to involve the child as much as possible with the final decision.

13.3.2 Blindness

Patients who are registered as partially sighted or blind are not excluded for screening. A patient may have some sight remaining and if deemed by an ophthalmologist that treatment for DR may retain some precious sight then a patient is eligible for screening. Only patients who have no perception of light in both eyes, which is irreversible, should be excluded from screening permanently.

13.3.3 Physical or mental disability

The presence of either a physical or a mental disability in patients does not infer exclusion from being screened; screening programmes must act under the regulations of the Disability Discrimination Act, and make every effort possible where mobility is an issue. Just because a patient cannot be digitally screened they may still be able to be screened by an ophthalmologist. Only when treatment (i.e. laser therapy) is impossible should a patient be excluded from screening. If an ophthalmologist decides that treatment would be impossible they should write to the screening scheme and the patient's GP and put the patient on either the temporary inactive list, with a review date detailed, or on the permanently inactive list.

13.3.4 Terminal illness

A person with diabetes who is terminally ill should continue being screened as long as the patient is capable and happy to do so. If treatment is possible, retaining sight could increase the quality of life for terminally ill patients. If the patient or GP makes an informed decision that treatment would be futile, then the patient should be placed either on the temporarily inactive list, and a re-assessment date decided, or on the permanently inactive list.

13.3.5 **Already in ophthalmology care for DR**

A patient who is currently being treated by an ophthalmologist for DR may be removed from the active list and put onto the temporary inactive list; a review date to monitor their status should be set. A yearly report of their DR grading should be sent to the screening scheme. If patients are discharged, they should be placed back on the active list.

13.3.6 **In ophthalmology care for other lesions**

A patient with diabetes who is in the care of an ophthalmologist for something other than DR should still be digitally screened annually. This is, however, unless the clinical lead has made an agreement with certain ophthalmologists/departments that screening is done during eye appointments. If this is the case then the patient should be removed from the active list and put on the temporary inactive list; a review date to monitor the status should be set. A yearly report of the DR grading should be sent to the screening scheme. If a patient is discharged he or she should be placed back onto the active list.

13.3.7 **Private patients**

Patients being screened or treated for DR outside the NHS screening scheme should still be invited to attend screening appointments and given the right to choose whether they would like an appointment.

13.3.8 **Patients in residential care or prisons**

Patients who are within residential care, such as those patients in nursing homes or prisons, should be treated in the same way as any other patients and only excluded from screening for other reasons stated above.

Summary

Effective administration is one of the keys to a successful screening programme, so that the correct subjects get an invitation, obtain an accurate quality assured screen, and receive timely results and treatment. Administration costs money and adequate funding may cause problems for screening programmes in the early years, including many schemes in our region. The DR screening programmes have clear guidance on who should be excluded. Our experience is that there are significant difficulties of organization within hospital eye services to allow a seamless pathway between screening and treatment to occur regardless of the nature of the chronic ophthalmological condition.

Chapter 14

Models of screening and IT

Andrew Mills

Key points

- Screening needs a central storage and computer, 'the server', to receive and serve data, including images, to users.
- At the point of use, one client PC collects for, or displays data from, the central unit.
- A secure transfer medium is required to communicate data between the client PC and the server.
- Image compression provides a useful tool to save storage space and improve response time for data transfers.
- Models of screening determine which transfer medium is most appropriate.

14.1 Introduction

For screening to work properly co-ordination is vital. Simply acquiring images in far-flung corners of a programme is of little use without a well-developed infrastructure to direct the care where it is needed. This infrastructure comes in the form of two key components: acquisition, movement, and review of data through the programme, 'The Model', and the Information Technology (IT) required for shuffling the data round the various components of the model. Both are interrelated and the needs of one must be balanced against the limitations of the other; and both must be balanced against the efficacy and cost of provision of the scheme. It is neither appropriate nor practical to enforce one model or one IT infrastructure on a retinal screening programme (Figure 14.1).

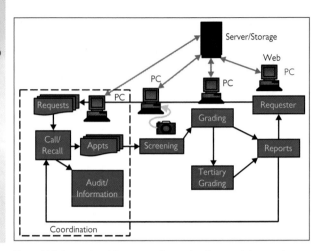

Figure 14.1 A typical workflow pattern showing data flow round the screening model. A hardware layer applied to this, indicates how the data flows backwards and forwards from the Server and PCs.

14.2 **IT and screening**

Image and data capture, image grading, data review, audit, and self-improvement are all completely possible without the need of a complicated IT infrastructure, and all the more complicated to coordinate practically without IT!

It is the job of IT to make the screening programme possible, and as far as possible to do so quietly in the background without interference. Properly done, it relieves the user of repetitive chores, incorrect information, and multiple data entry. The holy grail of any IT infrastructure is to enter the correct data only once. Sadly, in most instances this is not always possible, and in many cases incorrect implementation very often leads to unnecessary duplication of effort. Indeed, with data security a high priority, very often the various IT systems in the NHS are not directly interconnected and this leads to multiple re-entry of data, (the possibility for error), and almost certainly with frustration for the patient, not to mention those who administer the systems.

For the screening programme alone though, how can IT help? All models of screening will need to accumulate data centrally to ensure the needs of the patients, and the needs of the programme to monitor that the activities are being met. This central repository is a computer, known as a SERVER, connected to a large storage repository to hold the incoming images, and the database that will be used to manage the dataset that is needed to identify each patient, image, and image grade held on the system. From the central database, queries can be asked of the data, which allows the administrators of the screening programme to audit the processes involved and audit, address and correct any shortcomings. In the community, CLIENT computers (simple PCs) are used to collect and receive data from the server. Between the two lies a connection medium that depends on the model of the screening programme.

14.2.1 **The techie bit …**

Before discussing the screening programme models, and how they connect server to client, the technical bridge must be crossed; to fully understand how IT applies to screening requires some knowledge of the basic technologies.

14.2.2 **The anatomy of a personal computer**

A computer has several defined parts that make the whole, and these parts comprise the hardware (literally the stuff that can be touched!). From the largest super computer to the smallest hand-held, the basic anatomical structures of computers are unchanged. In the animal kingdom this is analogous to knowing that for mammals, there is a skeleton, brain, heart, and lungs, for example; but how they are packaged gives rise to the animal. In a computer there is a brain, the central processing unit (CPU), long-term storage (a hard disc or HD); short-term storage or working area (the memory, or RAM as it is known), and a display (the screen). To assist data entry there is a keyboard and pointing device (the mouse). Linking the components together is a series of wires (known as the bus), and, a connecting mechanism known as the universal serial bus (USB) which allows communication with the outside world. Computers need a clock to orchestrate the machine, commonly known as the speed of the machine and is measured in hertz (cycles per second). Typical clock speeds at the time of writing are 1 to 3 gigahertz (giga is 10^9 or 1 billion).

14.2.3 **In the beginning was the bit**

Computers are effectively large arrays of simple switches connected together. Just as a simple switch has two states (on or off) so do the internal switches or transistors of a computer. Numerically the on state is represented as the number 1 also known as a 'High', whilst the off position is represented by a zero (0), or 'Low'. By cascading switches together, a clever design can be created which, when triggered by the clock, allows complex calculations to be carried out; and for a computer to make decisions, there is a process known as running software. Software is a list of decision making instructions which the computer follows.

To store these states, we need a hardware called 'memory' (because it remembers the state it is set in) which is a location that can be updated and can hold onto the data without loss. The smallest piece of memory is the bit, and it stores just one piece of data, a high or a low. Memory requires power to operate; remove the power and it will 'forget' what is stored.

The Bit on its own would not offer much, but it does indicate that the best way to use a computer is to work in the binary base (by comparison humans are most effective using the decimal base, or numbers between 0 and 9). The most practical work unit of memory is the **byte**, which is a collection of 8 bits. Therefore each byte can contain 256 different variations of highs and lows (2 multiplied by itself 7 times, or 2^8).

To be really useful, several bytes are required to store information, so you will very often hear the terms kilobytes (KB), megabytes (MB), and gigabytes (GB) mentioned. In computing, because binary counting is used, kilo does not represent 1000 or 10^3, but is the closest number to 1000 achieved when 2 is raised to a power—1024, or 2^{10}. Similarly mega is a kilo squared or 2^{20}, or 1024 × 1024, whilst giga is a kilo cubed, 1024 × 1024 × 1024 or 2^{30}. Terabytes (TB) are the next level again, 2^{40}.

14.2.4 Computer memory—where the work is done

Computer memory is the scratchpad of a computer; all calculations and operations are held in memory whilst they are being used, and often it is described by the acronym RAM, meaning randomly accessed memory (i.e. the memory can be accessed in any order). Software is loaded into memory, and 'executed' (i.e. the processor loads each instruction in the program in turn and carries out the requests). Modern computers at the time of writing have between 512MB and 4GB of memory for program use. Very often there will be other memory in a computer dedicated for use by other parts of the system; for example, the graphics card (which is responsible for the screen display) will have dedicated memory.

Turn off a computer and the memory will be lost; it is said to be 'volatile', as it requires power to maintain the data residing in memory.

14.2.5 **Hard drive storage—the filing cabinet**

A hard drive, (or hard disc drive to be accurate) is the filing cabinet of the computer. Data are written to the hard disc for long-term storage, and unlike RAM, it is safely stored even when the power is off. Data are written to a magnetic surface using a writing 'head' which also doubles as the reading 'head'.

Hard disk drives are an extension of a technology where flat floppy plastic discs with a magnetized layer were used to contain data. These 'floppies' could not store much data, and because the read/write head actually contacted the surface, over time they wore out. A hard disc drive by comparison, consists of a spinning platter with a magnetized surface. The data can be stored, or written, as a series of magnetic changes on the hard disc, and read off again just as easily. The heads never touch the platter, but fly on a cushion of air about one thousandth the thickness of a human hair above the disc surface. As there is no contact, hard drives will not suffer from wear of the disk surface. To ensure that dust does not contaminate the surface and destroy the hard disc drive, the platter is contained within an hermetically sealed case. With a rigid structure, data can be written much more closely together and the capacity of a hard drive far exceeds that of its floppy cousin. Today, hard drives able to store 1TB of data are fairly common, and the computing industry expects data storage capability to rise by an order of magnitude within 5 years.

14.2.6 **The CPU**

The CPU is the heart of a computer. Every instruction to perform an operation is fed from memory to the CPU, and at the heart of every CPU are miniature transistors which switch between high and low states to make decisions; current CPUs have 550 million transistors on a sliver of silicon not much larger than your thumbnail; the wires between them are just 45nm wide (that is 1 millionth the thickness of a human hair). A CPU can perform mathematics, such as addition, subtraction, multiplication, and division; and it can make logical decisions using a branch of mathematics known as Boolean logic, as well as direct the data traffic round the computer. A CPU is 'clocked' or driven by a regular signal (hence the term 'clock'), at a high frequency. The frequency of the clock is often used as a measure of the speed of a computer, however clock speed alone is not a good indicator of this and indeed the current CPUs have clock speeds lower than the previous generation even though they are faster. Typical clock speeds at present are about 1.6 to 2.6GHz, or about the same frequency as the microwaves that heat up food!

14.2.7 **The operating system (OS)**

A computer is useless unless it has a commanding program to tell it what to do, and this is the job of the operating system (OS). The OS is a software (literally an entity which has no physical embodiment other than the media on which it is presented) program that handles all the input (mouse and keyboard, for example) and output (graphic display, sound, printing, etc.); other software programs run within an environment created by the OS and rely on the OS to provide interfaces to the hardware layers. Modern operating systems are complicated pieces of software which provide an environment with a common look and feel. Each time a mouse is moved, it is the job of the OS to move the mouse pointer on screen by a corresponding amount. At the same time in the background the OS is maintaining the computer, making sure the hard drive is ready to supply or receive data, the screen displays the correct information, and that programs are able to run in memory, accessing the correct memory locations and hardware as needed. You can think of an operating system as a very busy ringmaster in a circus, marshalling all the acts and keeping the show on schedule.

14.2.8 **Software**

Software programs are the tools we use on a computer to record data, number crunch, play games, and handle our way in the electronic world of e-mail and the World Wide Web. Retinal screening makes great use of software to coordinate the collection and processing of data. Data are collected in a structured file called a database, and a database manager controls the flow of the data into and out of the database. Imaging utilities enable the collection of data from digital cameras and allow manipulation on screen to obtain the best views of the underlying pathology. The end user knows this software simply by the software's name, but in reality this software has several component parts, from the software program on the client PC to the database manager and image storage software on the server.

14.3 **Images**

Of particular interest to the screening model is how a computer, and indeed a digital camera, handle images or pictures. Being digital devices, the camera and computer treat images as a grid of squares, each one containing an element of the image. These picture elements or 'pixels', simply contain a level of colour or grey; they do not contain any other information, such as shape. The more pixels in a given area of an image, the finer the resolution of the image will be. Typically the image from a digital camera will be in excess of 3000 pixels wide by 2000 pixels high—a total of six million pixels in the images. The current professional and semi-professional cameras have images in the region of 10–12 megapixels.

The number of pixels in an image is only part of the equation in describing an image digitally. Each pixel has to contain colour information and therefore a pixel has to consist of bytes to hold the colour information. As light is built up from three primary colours, red, green, and blue, each pixel uses three bytes to hold a value representing the intensity of one of the primary colours. With each byte capable of holding a value between 0 and 255 (256 different levels), a pixel therefore can hold 256^3 or 16 million colours.

To store a 6-megapixel image therefore requires three times the number of bytes, or 18 megabytes; if an image was stored in a one-to-one relationship. Fortunately, there are methods known as compression algorithms which enable an image to be considerably compressed and stored in a much smaller space.

14.3.1 Image compression

Compression algorithms are able to store information in a smaller space by a process known as tokenization, where repetitive phrases such as the word 'The' surrounded by spaces is replaced in a document by a token. A table at the head of the file is also created which stores the token against the phrase it replaces. There are over 300 'the' phrases in this chapter alone. So replacing this phrase with a single token would save over 1.2KB alone, as each letter removed saves one byte. To recreate the original document the token is replaced by the original phrase which results in the original document being restored exactly. Whilst this is a simplistic view of compression it does serve to illustrate the principle that a file on disk need not take up the space it occupies in memory, and introduces the concept of lossless compression, where an uncompressed file is exactly the same after undergoing compression/expansion as it was before the process.

Whilst it is possible to compress images using lossless compression, the amount of space saved although good is not huge. Typical reductions may at best be from 1.5–2.5 to 1, depending on the algorithm used. Much higher compression ratios can be achieved by using an algorithm which is not too careful about re-instating the exact equivalent of what was originally compressed. In textual terms, this is equivalent to compressing the phrase

'The Colour of Money'

And uncompressing it using the American spelling:

'The Color of Money'.

Contextually it is the same, but it is a likeness, not an exact duplicate. Extrapolating this concept to images results in an image reducing in size by almost 20 times and still uncompressing to a faithful replica of the original data. However, to achieve such impressive results means that data must be lost in the process, and it is called 'Lossy Compression'.

14.3.2 **The jpeg (or jpg) image**

There are several types of compression developed for different applications, and a whole host specifically for images, differing in the amount of compression available. The Joint Photographic Experts Group (JPEG) have defined a standard form of lossy compression which works particularly well with photographic images, where image data are built up of many infinitely varying shades, or hues, of colour of differing brightness. Jpeg compression yields high levels of compression (therefore small file sizes) for relatively small loss of image quality. Jpeg compression uses an algorithm that has some user definable parameters to control the level of compression. These parameters are often hidden from view in software programs and the user is simply asked a question to indicate how much compression is required, and is sometimes referred to as a quality factor.

Here the JPEG standard exploits the fact that the human eye does not see an image the way a digital camera records it. Particularly, the human eye is less responsive to changes in a colour shade than in brightness, and indeed there are many shades of colour that cannot be perceived; they appear identical to other shades to the human eye. Therefore by merging these shades the amount of information in an image can be reduced without affecting the overall quality of the image to the human eye. The actual method of reduction uses a complicated analysis based on a 16-pixel block and a mathematical technique known as a cosine transform. It is easier to think in these terms; rather than storing 256 levels of blue (1 byte's worth) that cannot be discerned, store 16 levels that can; therefore each image will occupy 1/16 the space because unnecessary information is not being stored.

It is very important to note that the image size, height, and width are not reduced in any way when an image is compressed, the original image and reproduction are the same size, and it is just the data within the image that is altered. It is our experience that a 500KB image is an acceptable file size with no loss of detail for grading.

14.3.3 **Just the right size?**

For the most part obtaining an image of the correct size is the domain of camera manufacturers and software suppliers to retinal screening, but it is always worth being aware of the consequences of compressing an image and recognizing the evidence of compression artefacts when an image has been over compressed.

To obtain a compressed image which obtains the best level of compression with no visible artefacts in the image is a fine balancing act, as seen in Figure 14.2. Under compression is not a problem, it simply results in a larger image, and there are no compression-induced artefacts in the image.

Over compression, however, can have serious consequences though; it may result in over emphasis of small normal variations of colour, by coalescing areas of similar colour into a more discernable shade. In properly compressed images, the coalescing of similar shades is between shades of colour that cannot be differentiated by the human eye. In over compressed images, the coalescing of shades will include shades that are further apart, and the subtle gradual shift of shades between colours starts to appear as a step change. In low over compression examples, artefacts of compression show up initially as subtle blocks in an image, usually in areas of broadly similar shades (e.g. the sky blue background in the holiday photos) as seen in Figure 14.3. Excessive over compression results in the blocks of colour joining together; repeated over the image it may look more like a series of colour contours than a true colour image, as in Figure 14.4.

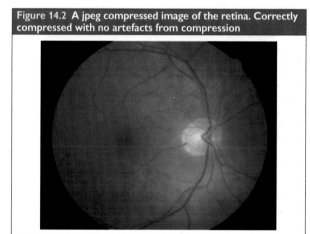

Figure 14.2 A jpeg compressed image of the retina. Correctly compressed with no artefacts from compression

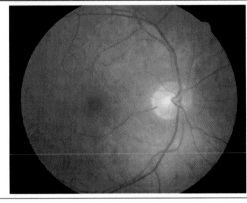

Figure 14.3 Over compression of the image from Figure 14.2. Notice the banding in the left-hand side of the image

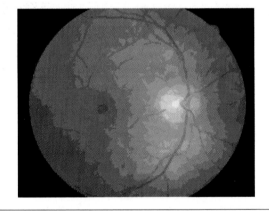

Figure 14.4 Extreme over compression. Image detail is lost as visible shades are merged into one common shade

14.3.4 **The right size**

Several papers have been written on acceptable levels of compression. However, as camera technologies improve, the number of pixels on the camera light sensor increases, and hence the natural size of an image rises, as will the compressed image size when compressed properly. At the time of writing, 12-megapixel images, or image sizes of 36mb before compression are not uncommon. Whereas 5 years earlier, a 5-megapixel image would have been seen as enormous. Therefore, compressing an image from bigger sensors by the same factor of compression will result in a compressed image that is also larger. Increasing the compression factor will reduce the image size, but will cause the compression artefacts to become more evident.

Interestingly, jpeg compression does not compress every image by the same degree, even if the original, uncompressed image size is the same. The amount of compression is dependent on the detail in the image to be manipulated. The more detail, the larger the image will be when compressed. It is only possible to indicate generally what compression levels are expected for a given type of image. The NSC workbook expects compression levels in the order of 20 to 1 to be applied for saving images to a hard drive, and more than this will lead to visible compression artefacts.

14.4 Screening models

Broadly, there are two extremes of models that lie at opposite ends of a spectrum of retinal screening models. The one starting point is the indirect approach, where remote screeners take images, collected locally on a computer and send in the data afterwards. At the other end lies the directly connected approach where data are transferred back and forth to a central location immediately (in IT parlance this is known as real-time) from the point of screening provision. Between these two extremes lie a number of provisions that may suit the retinal screening programme being considered. No one model is a perfect solution and several compromises may be needed along the way.

14.4.1 Model 1: remote data collection, 'The Man in the van' scenario

As discussed, rural locales demand a different approach to providing a retinal screening programme. A properly fitted van with camera, computer, and operator targeting specific locales on a regular basis can serve the needs of a population far more effectively than asking users to visit a screening centre many miles away. Here the operator takes photos and collects them on the local PC. How do we make sure that the data from the central call/recall centre are loaded on the PC in the van, and equally importantly the collected data are transferred back to the central server?

The solution is to have a messaging structure built into the software that governs data transfer between two systems, and governs upload and download of data to and fro. The local PC in the van is then treated as a miniature screening programme, and the one machine is its own server, image repository, database, and client application. Data can then be transferred from the PC when the van returns to its home location or when it reaches a suitable connection, the Internet/the NHSnet. Potentially, if enough security can be ensured, by utilizing Virtual Private Networks (VPNs) (where a private network is created on a public network, and appears to the user as a direct connection to the private network), the growing number of WiFi hotspots (areas which are served by a public wireless connection to the Internet) could be utilized to allow data transfer to occur when the van is parked near any location supporting a WiFi[1] cloud—the local café for instance! Patients turning up unannounced may have to be re-registered on the local system to be screened or turned away as the database will not contain a complete set of patient registrations, but simply the data required to screen the patients already stored.

14.4.2 Model 2: indirect remote locations

A halfway house between the man in the van and a direct connection, indirect remote locations are those whereby optometrists in the community are appointed to screen patients for the screening programme and possibly primary grade the images for the service. In this instance, the location can be thought of as a fixed location man in a van. Again the local PC is a miniature screening programme in its own right and again the data must be communicated to the central server by a messaging system. Similarly the use of the Internet and VPNs comes into play. Data are messaged back and forth securely along public lines to the central server. Again the problem of local registration raises its head.

14.4.3 Model 3: directly connected locations

Here the client PC is directly connected to the NHS net and can communicate directly with the server. The PC may be located in a GP's surgery or outreach clinic, or in an N3[2] connected optometrist's practice.[3] No messaging is required at this point and the information is never stored permanently on the local system. This model brings about some very different problems and some very important advantages to the screening program. Notably the data are pulled from the server in real time with images and grading data uploaded to the main server the instant they are collected. Here, it is possible to ensure that the idea of only having to enter patient registration data once is viable as far as the screening programme is concerned.

1 A wireless network in a public location, the cloud refers to the area in which a connection can be reliably established.

2 N3 is the third generation private NHS network designed to provide connection facilities at high speed between all NHS locales and agencies.

3 A PCT may employ an optometrist for the purposes of screening with a suitable contract; by supplying the PC to the screening locale and maintaining control over its security, the optometrist can be connected to N3 as an outreach locale under the terms of N3 security.

In addition, should there be an urgent need to review a patient by an ophthalmologist, the real-time nature of data transfer would allow this. Indeed, cross-pollination of ideas in this instance is much easier as a more experienced person can review images of a difficult patient whilst on the telephone to the grader grading the images, and pass on their experience directly.

14.4.4 **Data transfer**

Each screening model must transfer data from the client PC to the server and vice versa. To do this, either the database must create a message set and 'post' it to the server, receiving more data in return, or communicate in real time with the server along secure pathways. For secure transmission, the data must be encrypted such that no one can read the data easily, and this applies equally to the data held on a memory key or the data sent along a network cable.

A messaging solution can make use of any medium, from USB memory sticks, via optical storage, through to a VPN connection to the server, whilst the directly connected method must have a direct connection to the server using a network either along the N3 network or using a VPN connection to the server.

Each method has its advantage and disadvantage: optical media and USB memory sticks can be lost, corrupted, or damaged in transit; and it goes without saying that the data contained on the media must be encrypted to prevent information escaping in the event of a physical media loss. In their favour is the lack of need to be close to a network connection; useful if in remote locations too far away from a broadband connection (dial-up connections are useless in these situations as the amount of data to be transferred during the day could exceed 100 megabytes or more).

The direct connection model relies heavily on permanent stable connections to the server, something that is not always guaranteed as anyone with experience of such a system will tell you. And any faults will only ever occur on the busiest afternoon!

14.5 **Conclusions**

The models outline the major methodologies, together with advantages and pitfalls of each. No one method is king and in most cases, there is much to be gained from a combination of methods. An understanding of the IT infrastructure is integral to retinal screening, with the remote messaging to the direct connection model. When the IT system freezes and locks in clinical practice is when an understanding of the IT underlying becomes of major relevance.

Key references

Basu A, Kamal AD, Illahi W, Khan M, Stavrou P and Ryder RE. (2003). Is digital image compression acceptable within diabetic screening? *Diabetic Medicine*, **20**: 766–71.

UK National Screening Committee (August 2007).Essential Elements in Developing a Diabetic Retinopathy Screening Programme; Workbook 4: section 1.5.

www.jpeg.org

www.wikipedia.org Search for jpeg

Chapter 15

Training and accreditation for retinal screening

Margaret Clarke

Key points

- It is a requirement that all staff working in a national screening programme are appropriately trained for their role.
- A certificate in diabetic retinopathy screening (NVQ level 3), administered and awarded by City and Guilds, London, has been established.
- Of the eight major units of knowledge of the certificate there is the ability to claim Acquired Prior Experiential Learning (APEL), appropriate to previous experience and professional background
- A higher degree (MSc) has been developed at Warwick University.

15.1 Introduction

A requirement of the National Service Framework (NSF) for Diabetes is that all staff involved in a diabetic screening programme should be properly trained and accredited.

It stipulates that people with diabetes should be confident that any member of staff that they see

- Is properly trained and up to date
- Provides high quality care underpinned by clinical and service protocols and audit
- Has the interpersonal skills to communicate effectively with them.

Competences covering all the tasks involved in the identification of sight-threatening DR were developed with Skills for Health as part of the overall Diabetes Competence Framework. The retinopathy competences completed Four Nations (England, Wales, Scotland, and Northern Ireland) collaboration and were approved as National Occupational Standards in February 2005 (www.retinalscreening.co.uk or www.skillsforhealth.org.uk).

15.2 **Accreditation of competence**

A Level 3 Certificate in Diabetic Retinopathy Screening has been developed as an accreditation of the minimum level of competence required by ALL personnel involved in the identification of sight-threatening DR in the English National Screening Programme. Prior to the development of the certificate there was no qualification for diabetic retinal screeners and no regulation.

It is in acceptance of the need for accreditation in this evolving career that the certificate and further qualifications are being developed. Accreditation is a one-off measure of current competence. It recognizes that the learner has been assessed against the standards set for the profession and has achieved the required standard. Principally, it is designed to protect the patient but also protects the worker and employer. Ultimately it is hoped it will encourage the recruitment and retention of staff. It is not a measure of continuing competence; rather continuing competence is achieved through continuing professional development and is measured by performance indicators (internal and external quality assurance) in the National Screening Programme and appraisal.

15.3 **The Certificate in Diabetic Retinopathy Screening**

This qualification is a vocationally related qualification (VRQ) which has been developed by a multidisciplinary reference group comprising of subject experts from the UK Four Nations and educationalists.

City and Guilds in London are the awarding body for this qualification, and candidates are registered and certified through them.

The award comprises of the following:

1. Three mandatory units and three optional units
- Learners will need to achieve six units in order to achieve the full qualification
- Learners will be advised to take units that reflect their job role
- Learners will be able to take additional units as required.

Certificates of unit credit will be issued to learners who are successful in one or more units, but who do not necessarily wish to complete the whole programme.

The mandatory units are as follows:
- Unit 1: National Screening Programmes, Principles, Processes and Protocols. 30 Notional learning hours (NLH)
- Unit 2: Diabetes and its Relevance to Retinopathy Screening (30 NLH)

- Unit 3: Anatomy, Physiology and Pathology of the Eye and its Clinical Relevance (60 NLH).

The optional units are as follows:
- Unit 4: Preparing the Patient for Retinopathy Screening (20 NHL)
- Unit 5: Measuring Visual Acuity and Performing Pharmacological Dilatation (30 NLH)
- Unit 6: Imaging the Eye for the Detection of Diabetic Retinopathy (60 NLH)
- Unit 7: Detecting Retinal Disease (60 NLH)
- Unit 8: Classifying Diabetic Retinopathy (20 NLH)
- Unit 9: Administration and Management Systems in a Retinopathy Screening Programme (60 NLH).

Each unit has been assessed as requiring a specific number of hours to complete them, expressed as notional learning hours (NLH). However, it is our experience that well-qualified candidates need significantly less than the notional time to complete each unit.

It is clear that a number of different disciplines are likely to be involved in different diabetic retinopathy screening programmes, with different skill mix, for example, coordinators, administrators, photographers, and optometrists. To facilitate appropriate training, different occupational groups may do a number of appropriate units that are each accredited. Equally, some professional groups may already have competencies and training relevant to DR screening, for example, optometrists. Typical advice for optometrists is that they will not be required to complete assignments for the following units on production of appropriate evidence of Acquired Prior Experiential Learning (APEL) for units 3, 4, and 5.

Other candidates who have previous qualifications should contact the awarding centre for details since certain units may be available to the APEL process. However, candidates should be aware that to have APEL out of an individual unit may be costlier than taking the accreditation. Each unit can be individually certificated or a candidate can enrol for the whole award. Additional units must be taken by candidates if their job role extends beyond the six units in the award.

The following units are the minimum recommended for the various job roles in a screening programme for DR:
- Measurement of visual acuity (VA) and drop instillation: Units 1, 2, 4, and 5
- Imaging the eye: Units 1, 2, 3, 4, 5, and 6
- Grading DR (disease/no disease only): Units 1, 2, 3, and 7
- Grading DR (full disease grading): Units 1, 2, 3, 7, and 8
- Screening centre managers and administrators: Units 1, 2, 4, and 9.

15.4 **Higher qualifications**

A higher qualification for advancing knowledge and qualifications for retinal screeners has been developed. This acknowledges and supports the new career path and expertise of the DR screening workforce.

A Masters level degree in DR screening has been developed according to the principles of the degree.

Masters degrees are awarded to students who show

1. A systematic understanding of knowledge, and a critical awareness of current problems and/or new insights

2. A comprehensive understanding of techniques applicable to their own research or advanced scholarship

3. Originality in the application of knowledge

4. Conceptual understanding that enables the student to evaluate critically current research and to evaluate methodologies and develop critiques.

This higher qualification should allow appropriate personnel to develop and expand their portfolio to access higher NHS point scales (see Warwick University MSc prospectus).

Useful resources

A frequently asked questions document about the Certificate in Diabetic Retinopathy Screening & National Screening Programme for Diabetic Retinopathy Workbook (2007).

http://www.nscretinopathy.org.uk

http://www.drscertificate.org

http://www.cityandguilds.com

Chapter 16

Medical management of diabetic retinopathy

Paul M Dodson

> **Key points**
>
> - Medical management is focused on the proven benefit of tight glucose and blood pressure control.
> - Standard management includes multiple cardiovascular risk factor management with angiotensin receptor blockade, statin and fibrate treatment in addition to aspirin.
> - Targets to achieve include HbA1c <7%, blood pressure <140/80, and serum cholesterol <4mmol/l.
> - A number of new trials have demonstrated the beneficial effects on diabetic retinopathy (DR) of fenofibrate (lipid lowering), and Ruboxistaurin® (protein kinase C inhibition) with reduction of laser treatment and protection of vision.
> - A landmark study of an angiotensin receptor blocker is due to complete shortly (DIRECT study) which will provide data on the potential benefit of this treatment on both primary and secondary prevention of DR.

16.1 Clinical need

One of the most feared complications of diabetes is blindness and loss of vision. There has therefore been extensive clinical and laboratory research to target this complication, and progress has been made. Although the retinal leakage may be influenced by medical treatment, once capillary closure and ischaemia are extensive then medical therapies may have less impact. This is also the case when there is significant macula ischaemia and visual loss, such that retinal laser is contraindicated, and standard medical therapy is ineffective. Ischaemic maculopathy, therefore, remains a common cause of untreatable blindness in diabetic subjects. The basic management of type 1 and 2 diabetes is outlined in Chapter 1.

16.2 **Conventional risk factor modification**

16.2.1 **Glycaemia and blood pressure**

To achieve optimal glycaemic control requires the input of a multidisciplinary team to provide education and motivation for the diabetic patient. This will include general practitioners in close collaboration with other members of the healthcare team, including the practice and diabetes specialist nurses, dietitian, chiropodist, and psychologist (where appropriate), as well as the diabetes specialist care team.

The UKPDS (United Kingdom Prospective Diabetes Study), and the DCCT (Diabetes Control and Complications Trial) have confirmed beyond question the benefit of improving glycaemic control in both type 1 and 2 diabetics. Both these studies achieved a target glycated haemoglobin of around 7% (a measure of average glucose control over a 6 to 8 week period) with major reductions in microvascular complications. Of importance is the fact that any reduction in glycated haemoglobin was of benefit and that there was no threshold effect.

The DCCT trial in type 1 diabetics demonstrated that intensive insulin treatment achieving a 2% difference in glycosylated haemoglobin resulted in a 76% reduction of developing new retinopathy. Similarly in the UKPDS study in type 2 diabetics, for every 1% reduction in glycosylated haemoglobin translated into a 37% reduction of microvascular complications (see Figure 16.1). The reduced ocular microvascular endpoints were progression of diabetic retinopathy, laser requirement, and cataract.

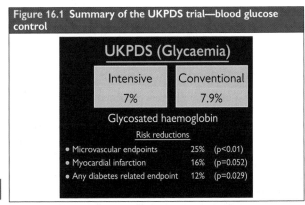

Figure 16.1 Summary of the UKPDS trial—blood glucose control

UKPDS (Glycaemia)

Intensive	Conventional
7%	7.9%

Glycosated haemoglobin

Risk reductions

• Microvascular endpoints	25%	(p<0.01)
• Myocardial infarction	16%	(p=0.052)
• Any diabetes related endpoint	12%	(p=0.029)

16.2.2 **Blood pressure control**

Tight control of blood pressure is also crucial as has been demonstrated in many large treatment trials. The UKPDS specifically studied microvascular endpoints, showing a 37% reduction in type 2 diabetics achieving a systolic blood pressure of 144mmHg at 7 years follow-up (see Figure 16.2), and 34% reduction in the proportion of patients with deterioration of retinopathy severity. The risk of microvascular complications was reduced by 11% per 10mmHg decrease in systolic blood pressure.

The preferred agents for treatment of hypertension in diabetes are as follows:

- ACE inhibitors or angiotension receptor blockers
- Thiazide diuretics
- Calcium channel blockers.

Almost all people with diabetes will require a combination of blood pressure-lowering drugs to achieve recommended targets, but some will require three or more. This combination is likely to include an ACE inhibitor or angiotensin receptor blockers (ARB) in view of their specific effects described in the following section.

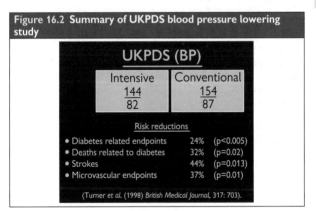

Figure 16.2 Summary of UKPDS blood pressure lowering study

UKPDS (BP)

	Intensive	Conventional
	144	154
	82	87

Risk reductions

• Diabetes related endpoints	24%	(p<0.005)
• Deaths related to diabetes	32%	(p=0.02)
• Strokes	44%	(p=0.013)
• Microvascular endpoints	37%	(p=0.01)

(Turner et al. (1998) British Medical Journal, 317: 703).

16.2.3 Angiotensin receptor blockade

The ARB are gaining more trial evidence of benefit, particularly in nephropathy, and are now being widely used. Evidence for renin-angiotensin system blockade is strongest for nephroprotection (kidney disease). A role for angiotensin has been suggested in in vitro experiments in retinal angiogenesis and tested in people with diabetes. The EURODIAB Controlled Trial of Lisinopril in Insulin-Dependent Diabetes (EUCLID) study suggested the potential of specific treatment of ACE inhibition (lisinopril) to diabetic retinopathy with 45% reduction of progression, but the study conclusion was confounded by better glucose control in the lisinopril group compared to control.

- A large randomized landmark trial of an ARB (candesartan) in 5231 diabetic patients is due to complete in 2008 (Diabetic REtinopathy Candesartan Trial—DIRECT study) which will provide data on whether there is benefit in both primary and secondary prevention of diabetic retinopathy in type 1 diabetics, and secondary prevention in type 2 patients. This will give the first data to identify whether ARB will have an effect on delaying the development of the first signs of DR (i.e. primary prevention).

Whilst it is clear that the effects of increasing blood pressure and glycaemic control are risk factors for microvascular disease, importantly these are **additive**, as shown in recent analysis from the UKPDS study and illustrated in Figure 16.3.

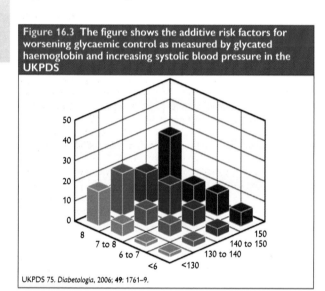

Figure 16.3 The figure shows the additive risk factors for worsening glycaemic control as measured by glycated haemoglobin and increasing systolic blood pressure in the UKPDS

UKPDS 75. *Diabetologia*, 2006; **49**: 1761–9.

16.2.4 **Lipid-lowering therapy**
Statin therapy has been proven to reduce cardiovascular (CV) disease in diabetic patients in both primary and secondary prevention, such that most type 2 diabetics should be on this group of drugs unless there is a contraindication or drug intolerance. Fibrate agents are widely used for treatment of predominantly increased triglyceride levels commonly in association with low high-density lipoprotein (HDL) cholesterol levels, but have less effect on cardiovascular disease in type 2 diabetics than statins.

More recently, data have confirmed that increasing total cholesterol and low-density lipoprotein (LDL) levels, as well as increasing fasting serum triglycerides, are associated with a greater risk of developing maculopathy and macula oedema (see Chapter 4, Figure 4.11).

The Collaborative Atorvastatin Diabetes Study (CARDS) assessed the effectiveness of atorvastatin 10mg daily versus placebo for primary prevention of CV events in patients with type 2 diabetes. Over 4 years, the results from CARDS demonstrated a trend towards reduction of laser therapy undertaken in the atorvastatin arm by 21%, but this did not reach statistical significance, and there was no influence on diabetic retinopathy progression. Thus the influence of statins on DR remains debatable, but if there is an effect, it is likely to be small.

The Fenofibrate Intervention and Event Lowering in Diabetes (FIELD) study, a large randomized trial designed to study the effects of the oral fibrate agent fenofibrate 200mg/day compared with placebo included the evaluation of microvascular endpoints. There was a highly significant 30% reduction in laser eye treatment in diabetic patients previously treated with fenofibrate. First laser treatment for macula oedema was reduced by 31% and for proliferative retinopathy by 30%. Whilst there was no effect on primary prevention, those patients with pre-existing retinopathy at entry to the trial benefited most, that is, in secondary prevention.

The ACCORD-EYE study, which is currently well underway, should allow further resolution of these issues. The ACCORD-EYE study has been designed to assess the effects of the ACCORD medical treatment strategies of tight control of glycaemia and blood pressure and management of dyslipidaemia on the course of DR in patients with type 2 diabetes. Specifically, it will address whether a treatment strategy using a fibrate and a statin reduces the development and progression of DR compared with one using placebo and a statin.

16.2.5 **Aspirin**

Diabetic patients with DR should be taking aspirin therapy, not because of a beneficial effect on diabetic retinopathy but because of the benefit of this agent comprising reduction in cardiovascular disease events in patients with DR, which was demonstrated some years ago in the ETDRS study of laser treatment. Aspirin could be associated with increased haemorrhage which could be deleterious to DR, particularly with fragile new vessel formation in proliferative retinopathy. However, trials of this potential effect have not shown any deleterious effect on retinal and vitreous haemorrhage.

16.3 **Multifactorial interventions**

The clinical trial evidence for treatment benefit for diabetic microvascular disease is largely based on single risk factor interventions. However, the Steno 2 study has provided some data on the benefits of a multifactorial intervention programme. Type 2 diabetics were randomly allocated to an intensive treatment programme of drugs targeting glycaemia, blood pressure lowering, and lipid lowering, in addition to specific treatment with ACE inhibition, statins, and aspirin. Over a 7.8-year period, there was a large benefit in reduction of cardiovascular disease endpoints by 53%, diabetic nephropathy by 61%, and DR progression by 58%. However, there was still progression of diabetic retinopathy in 25% of patients despite intensive treatment, hence the concept of residual risk. The benefit was also maintained on longer term follow-up.

The management guidelines used in the Steno 2 study is the current therapeutic approach advised for patients with diabetes. This approach does require considerable poly pharmacy and multiple drugs, but more combinations of commonly used drugs are becoming available.

16.4 **New potential therapies for DR**

There are five main chemical pathways implicated in the pathogenesis of diabetic microvascular complications:

- Increased polyol pathway flux
- Increased advanced glycation end product (AGE) formation
- Activation of the protein kinase C (PKC) isoforms
- Increased hexosamine pathway flux
- Increased angiogenic growth factors, for example, VEGF, growth hormone, and angiotensins.

Specific inhibitors of each of these pathways have been tested as shown in Figure 16.4, which combine the vascular changes as well as the metabolic pathways leading to the retinal leakage and ischaemia, fundamental to development of DR.

The first therapeutic approach tested in large clinical trials was of aldose reductase inhibitors (e.g. ranirestat). This group of drugs blocks the accumulation of excess intracellular sorbitol derived in the presence of hyperglycaemia. The retinal studies demonstrated a weak effect of these drugs on microaneurysm formation, but had an unfavourable side effect profile, and so have not been adopted for clinical use.

More recent emphasis has been placed in human trials of DR on newer agents. These have included the PKC inhibitors (Ruboxistaurin®), growth factor inhibition (growth hormone and insulin-like growth factor (IGF)-1, lipid lowering (see Section 16.2.4), and ARB (see Section 16.2.3).

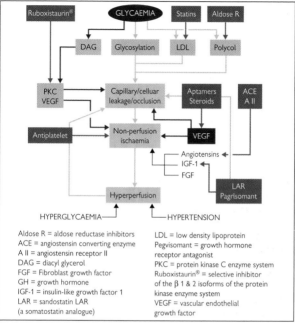

Figure 16.4 Pathogenetic mechanisms in the development of DR. The two major mechanisms of vascular changes—hyperglycaemia and hypertension—and the biochemical pathways implicated in the pathogenesis of DR are illustrated.

There is great interest in the use of intra-vitreal anti-VEGF therapy which is licensed for use in treatment of age-related macula degeneration; but these agents are now undergoing human trials in patients with DR. These are outlined in Chapter 17, but will be reserved for patients with more advanced retinopathy rather than for early medical treatment or prevention of development.

16.4.1 Growth hormone antagonism

Prior to the widespread availability of retinal laser treatment, pituitary ablation was a treatment option for proliferative retinopathy, based on a case report of a young woman whose proliferative DR resolved after post-partum infarction of her pituitary gland. A natural inhibitor of growth hormone action is somatostatin. The development of somatostatin analogues that could be given by injection two to four weekly allowed for this treatment to be tested. Two large randomized trials of growth hormone antagonism using a somatostatin analogues have been recently completed and they reported an inconclusive result with no clear effect on the progression of pre-proliferative DR. Previous pilot studies had also suggested that this therapeutic approach may also be beneficial in treating aggressive proliferative retinopathy, but this has not to date been explored in large clinical trials.

16.4.2 PKC enzyme inhibition

Protein Kinase C (PKC) is an enzyme activated by hyperglycaemia-induced synthesis of diacyl glycerol I, resulting in increased VEGF levels and consequently, exudation from the retinal vessels. There are 12 isoforms of the PKC enzyme, but it is the PKC-β_2 isoform that is preferentially activated in the tissues involved in diabetic microvascular damage, particularly the retina. Specific activation of PKC-β_2 increases retinal vascular permeability and neovascularization in animal models.

A novel drug, Ruboxistaurin® has been identified, which specifically blocks the PKC-β_2 isoform and which in animal studies, reduces retinal oedema and neovascularization in diabetic animals. Initial results in human studies supported these observations. The recent randomized, placebo-controlled, Phase III PKC-β Inhibitor Diabetic Retinopathy Study (PKC–DRS2) study has examined the potential of this new drug in 685 patients with diabetes, randomized to either placebo or 32mg/day oral Ruboxistaurin® for a 3-year treatment period.

The trial demonstrated that Ruboxistaurin® treatment resulted in a clinically and statistically significant decrease in visual loss as well as a reduction in laser treatment, with most benefit in those with moderate to severe pre-proliferative retinopathy. A summary of the key results is shown in Box 16.1.

Additionally, the safety profile of Ruboxistaurin® has shown no concerns and no real adverse effects; indeed, in this study the mortality rate was shown to be less in the Ruboxistaurin® group compared with placebo. Ruboxistaurin® has an approvable letter from the Food and Drugs Administration (FDA), and trials are ongoing.

Box 16.1 Principal results in the Diabetic Retinopathy Study (DRS-2)

Ruboxistaurin® led to

- 41% reduction in sustained visual loss
- 30% reduction in first application of laser
- Effects which were apparent after 9–12 months of Ruboxistaurin® treatment
- No difference in progression of DR between Ruboxistaurin® and placebo.

16.5 **Other therepeutic approaches**

Two other pathways have been investigated in an attempt to prevent and ameliorate diabetic microvascular disease. The first is non-enzymatic protein glycation resulting in the formation of advanced glycolysation end products (AGEs), which accumulate in life and are increased in diabetes. AGE modifications have serious consequences for macromolecular function, especially in the case of DNA, important structural proteins, enzymes, and growth factors. The first blocker of this pathway was aminoguanidine which demonstrated prevention of development of DR in dogs, but the drug had unwanted side effects. Other related AGE inhibitors may eventually find a place in the management of diabetes mellitus.

The second pathway is the increased free radical formation and oxidative stress in diabetic subjects which have a plausible mechanism of injury. However, clinical trials of anti-oxidants, vitamin C, or vitamin E, have been largely disappointing.

Summary

The medical management of patients with DR is focused on the proven benefit of tight glucose and blood pressure control, with multiple cardiovascular risk factor intervention with ACE inhibition, statin and fibrate treatment in addition to aspirin. The study of abnormal
biochemical pathways and increased angiogenic growth factors has led to a number of new potential treatments, including intra-vitreal anti-VEGF agents, and PKC blockade.

Further reading

Brownlee M (2001). Biochemistry and molecular cell biology of diabetic complications. *Nature*, **414**: 813–20.

Chowdhury TA, Hopkins D, Dodson PM, *et al.* (2002).The role of serum lipids in exudative diabetic maculopathy: is there a place for lipid lowering therapy? *Eye*, **16**: 689–93.

Clarke M and Dodson PM (2007). PKC inhibition and diabetic microvascular complications. *Best Practice and Research Clinical Endocrinology*, **21**(4): 573–86.

Colhoun HM, Betteridge DJ, Durrington PN, *et al.* Primary prevention of cardiovascular disease with atorvastatin in type 2 diabetes in the Collaborative Atorvastatin Diabetes (2004). *Lancet,* **364**: 685–69.

Diabetes Control and Complications Trial Group (1993). The effect of intensive treatment of diabetes on the development and progression of long-term complications in insulin-dependent diabetes mellitus. *New England Journal of Medicine*, **329**: 977–86.

Dodson P (2008). Medical treatment for diabetic retinopathy: do the FIELD microvascular study results support a role for lipid lowering. *Practical Diabetes Int*, **25**(2): 76–9.

Donaldson M and Dodson PM (2003). Medical treatment of diabetic retinopathy. *Eye*, **17**: 550–62.

The EUCLID Study Group (1997). Randomised placebo-controlled trial of lisinopril in normotensive patients with insulin-dependent diabetes and normoalbuminuria or microalbuminuria. *Lancet*, **349**: 1787–92.

Ferris FL 3rd, Davis MD, Aiello LM (1999). Treatment of diabetic retinopathy. *New England Journal of Medicine*, **341**: 667–8.

Gaede P, Vedel P, Larsen N, *et al.* (2003). Multifactorial intervention and cardiovascular disease in people with type 2 diabetes. *New England Journal of Medicine*, **348**: 383–93 (and **358**: 580–91, (2008)).

JBS 2: Joint British Societies' Guidelines on prevention of cardiovascular disease in clinical practice. *Heart*, **91**(suppl V): 1–52.; 2005.

Keech AC, Mitchell P, Summanen PA, *et al.*, for the FIELD study investigators (2007). Effect of fenofibrate on the need for laser treatment for diabetic retinopathy (FIELD study): a randomised controlled trial. *Lancet*, **370**(9600): 1687–97. Epub. 2007 Nov. 7.

Nguyen QD, Tatlipinar S, Shah SM, *et al.* (2006). Vascular endothelial growth factor is a critical stimulus for diabetic macular edema. *American Journal of Ophthalmology*; **142**: 961–969.

The PKC-DRS Study Group (2005). The effect of Ruboxistaurin® on visual loss in patients with moderately severe to very severe non-proliferative diabetic retinopathy. Initial results of the protein kinase C beta inhibitor retinopathy study (PKC-DRS) multicenter randomized clinical trial. *Diabetes*, **54**: 2188–97.

Sheetz MJ and King GL (2002). Molecular understanding of hyperglycaemia's adverse effects for diabetic complications. *Journal of American Medical Association*, **288**: 2579–88.

Sjolie AK, Porta M, Parving HH, *et al.* (2005). The DIabetic REtinopathy Candersartan Trials (DIRECT) Programme Renin Angiotensin Aldosterone System, **6**(1): 25–32.

Study (CARDS): multicentre randomized placebo-controlled trial. *Lancet*, 2004; **364**: 685–96.

UK Prospective Diabetes Study (UKPDS) Group (1998). Intensive blood-glucose control with sulphonylureas or insulin compared with conventional treatment and risk of complications in patients with type 2 diabetes (UKPDS 33). *Lancet*, 1998; **352**: 837–53.

UK Prospective Diabetes Study (UKPDS) Group (1998).Tight blood pressure control and risk of macrovascular and microvascular complications in type 2 diabetes: UKPDS 38. *British Medical Journal*, **317**: 703–13.

Chapter 17

Ophthalmic treatment of diabetic retinopathy

Jonathan M Gibson

Key points

- Laser photocoagulation remains the main treatment for diabetic retinopathy (DR).
- Laser photocoagulation is unlikely to improve vision once it has decreased but is effective in stabilizing vision.
- Treatment with intra-vitreal drugs for maculopathy is a major development.
- Optical coherence tomography is an invaluable new imaging tool for DR.
- Pars plana vitrectomy is available for advanced DR.

17.1 Ophthalmic treatment

The optimal treatment of diabetic retinopathy (DR) requires management of the underlying diabetes and related risk factors and ophthalmic treatments to preserve vision. Inevitably patients are generally best managed if there is close liaison between the treating ophthalmologist and the diabetic physician, and this is being increasingly facilitated in both diabetic and eye clinics by access to digital fundal images.

The management of DR is undergoing continuous evolution and the current strategies for preservation of vision in diabetic patients are summarized in the following sections. For an excellent overview, the reader is recommended to visit the *Royal College of Ophthalmologists Guidelines* (2005).

- Retinal laser treatment which is used for proliferative diabetic retinopathy (PDR) and maculopathy in different strategies
- Administration of anti-VEGF (vascular endothelial growth factor) agents either by peri-ocular or intra-ocular injection
- Treatment for advanced diabetic retinal disease by pars plana vitrectomy
- Treatment of patients with cataract with phacoemulsification and intra-ocular lens implantation.

161

The ophthalmologist has an important educational role by feedback of patients' findings and progress to the referring screening programme and to referring general practitioners, diabetic physicians, and optometrists. In this manner, the whole service benefits by a two-way flow of information to allow optimal medical and ophthalmological management.

17.2 **Retinal laser treatment**

Retinal lasers are widely available in ophthalmic departments and the vast majority of treatments are performed on an outpatient basis using a slit lamp with a laser attachment. A special contact lens is applied to the patient's cornea after local anaesthesia drops are instilled, and this allows a stereoscopic view to be obtained of the fundus. Different lenses are available for treatment of maculopathy and pan-retinal photocoagulation (PRP), depending on the angle of view and magnification required. An additional benefit of the lenses is that they very effectively help to control inadvertent movement of the patient's eye.

The commonest retinal laser available is the argon laser which in its original form produced two peaks of light in the blue-green and green part of the spectrum; but these have been superseded by green-only lasers emitting light in the band of 514nm, which are safer for use in the macular region and may be safer for the operator.

With advances in technology, the earlier gas lasers are now being replaced by solid state laser machines which are based on diode laser technology. This means they are considerably more robust and energy efficient than the earlier models and are extremely compact and portable. This latter point is important for cases that may be treated in outpatients as well as the operating theatre.

The latest advances have been the introduction of micropulse laser technology in which the retinal laser reactions are kept to a minimum to avoid collateral damage to healthy functioning retina and thereby lessen visual loss from laser treatment. Advances have also been made in the use of pattern application of laser burns by which multiple laser reactions in the retina set to a pre-determined pattern are achieved by a single application. This is the basis of new semi-automated retinal patterned scanning laser (PASCAL Photocoagulator, Optimedica) (Figure 17.1).

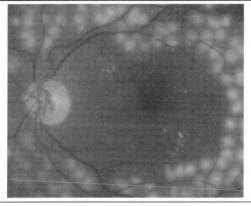

Figure 17.1 Fresh scatter laser PRP reactions after laser photocoagulation with 532nm frequency doubled YAG laser. Note the NVD

17.3 **Treatment for proliferative retinopathy**

Laser PRP for DR is an extremely important and effective treatment for sight preservation in PDR and this has been confirmed in a number of trials.

The Diabetic Retinopathy Study (DRS) was an important landmark trial that provides the main evidence base for laser treatment to PDR. The DRS was a prospective multicentre clinical trial which showed that scatter laser photocoagulation (PRP) reduced the risk of severe visual loss by at least 50%. It also confirmed that argon laser and xenon light coagulation were equally effective, but that harmful effects were more common with the old xenon machines, and this led to the widespread introduction of modern argon laser facilities into eye departments.

Scatter laser or PRP is indicated for PDR when new vessels in the retina (NVE) or new vessels on the optic disc (NVD) are present and are considered at risk of bleeding. The aim of PRP is to destroy the areas where there is capillary non-perfusion and retinal ischaemia. In most eyes, this will mean an application of over 2000 retinal burns of spot size 500 microns or more if the burns are smaller. It is usual practice in most units to fractionate this treatment into two sessions, which is more comfortable for the patient and is less associated with side effects. In this way treatment sessions are able to be completed in about 10–15 minutes (Figure 17.2).

Side effects of PRP:

1. Laser PRP can be uncomfortable for the patient and this is dependent on the duration and power of the laser burns, the amount given, the position in the fundus, and the wavelength of the laser energy. Most new lasers allow much shorter exposures to be given than in the conventional DRS and Early Treatment Diabetic Retinopathy Study (ETDRS) trial parameters, whilst still being effective, and generally nowadays there is no reason for laser PRP to be uncomfortable for most patients.

2. Vitreous haemorrhage may occur after laser PRP if there are extensive fronds of NVE present, and this is thought to be due to contraction and bleeding from the fronds.

3. Worsening of macular oedema following laser PRP is well recognized and is thought to occur as a decompensation of the macular capillaries probably due to alteration in macula blood flow. It can be prevented by fractionating laser PRP to smaller numbers of burns, by performing laser treatment for maculopathy before PRP and increasingly by the use of anti-VEGF intra-vitreal injections before or after laser PRP.

4. Inadvertent foveal burn may occur if there is sudden uncontrolled patient movement during laser treatment or if the operator becomes disorientated with fundus landmarks. It is usually a catastrophic event for the patient, and operator,

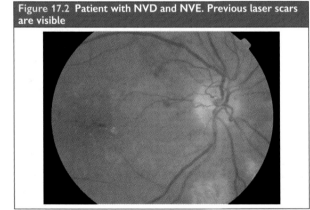

Figure 17.2 Patient with NVD and NVE. Previous laser scars are visible

giving rise to immediate and permanent loss of central vision. It is fortunately extremely rare and most ophthalmic units would never encounter a case but it is wise to be constantly aware of its possibility.

5. Loss of peripheral vision and reduction in night-time vision may occur if extensive PRP is given. This may have important implications for the patient if they are motor vehicle drivers, particularly if it is required as part of their employment. It may be a necessary risk for the patient to accept this as a means of maintaining the central vision, but it should be discussed with the patient prior to PRP being carried out. With newer laser technology and less collateral damage this is less common than in previous years when very heavy peripheral laser was given.

17.4 **Managing diabetic maculopathy**

The ETDRS was a large, prospective multicentre clinical trial which has shown that prompt laser treatment of clinically significant macular oedema (CSMO) can reduce the risk of visual loss by 50%. It also showed that visual improvement was unlikely, but that laser treatment was effective in preventing further visual loss.

CSMO is a useful concept for the management of diabetic maculopathy and is best detected and evaluated using slit lamp bio-microscopy with a Volk handheld lens or by a fundus contact lens. CSMO was defined by the ETDRS as the following:

• Retinal thickening at or within 500 microns of the centre of the macula (i.e. fovea)

• Hard exudates at or within 500 microns of the macula centre, if associated with thickening of the adjacent retina

• Retinal thickening of at least one disc area in extent, any part of which is within 1 disc diameter (DD) of the macular centre.

Optical coherence tomography has now become an indispensible tool in monitoring macular oedema.

17.4.1 **Methods of imaging the macula**

Fluorescein angiography is unnecessary for most cases of diabetic maculopathy and is not required for straightforward cases of focal macular oedema with circinate exudates rings. It is very useful once the diagnosis and decision to treat macular oedema have been made, as a guide to laser treatment. It is particularly important in those cases of ischaemic maculopathy where there may be perifoveal capillary hypoperfusion because in these cases laser photocoagulation may compromise remaining capillary circulation. It is also helpful in cases undergoing serial laser treatment that appear to be non-responsive.

Optical coherence tomography (OCT) has revolutionized the management of diabetic maculopathy. It is a non-invasive technique of visualizing the cross-section of the retina and allows the thickness of the retina and associated oedema to be measured and visualized. As it is non-invasive, it can be performed easily and quickly on patients and is particularly useful in monitoring the response to laser treatment and anti-VEGF injection for diabetic maculopathy (Figure 17.3).

17.4.2 Laser photocoagulation

The cumulative evidence to date indicates that photocoagulation therapy remains the mainstay of therapy for sight-threatening diabetic macular oedema. Based on the evidence of the ETDRS and previous less extensive studies, the following recommendations for the laser treatment of diabetic macular oedema, as identified as retinal thickening by clinical stereoscopic viewing on bio-microscopy or by stereoscopic fundus photographs, are proposed.

Laser therapy for maculopathy is recommended

1. where the centre of the macula is involved in which vision is 6/9 or less.

Laser treatment may be considered

2. only after counselling with regard to potential side effects and risks of treatment for patients in patients where vision is 6/6 or better. Laser therapy should involve scatter treatment in the area of leaking lesions 500 microns or more distant from the centre of the macula. Where there are no discrete identified lesions, that is, where leakage is diffuse, a grid of laser therapy should be applied. Areas of leakage may be identified by fluorescein angiography.

Generally, treatment for diabetic maculopathy is divided into focal laser burns, for localized retinal thickening, or a grid of laser burns avoiding the foveal avascular zone, for patients with diffuse macular oedema. Laser burns are titrated to produce a very gentle burn reaction as high energy burns may cause haemorrhage, choroidal neovascular membrane formation, or epiretinal membrane. Typical laser settings would be spot size 100 microns, duration 0.05 second, and power of 0.1–0.2mWatts (Figure 17.4).

It is still not obvious how focal laser treatment works but it is thought that it is either effective by direct treatment and closure of leaking microaneurysms or by an effect on the retinal pigment epithelium, and the outer blood retina barrier. This forms the basis of a recognised type of laser strategy called the 'modified grid'.

Figure 17.3 OCT scan of patient with macular oedema before and after intra-vitreal triamcinolone (a steroid) showing reduction in oedema

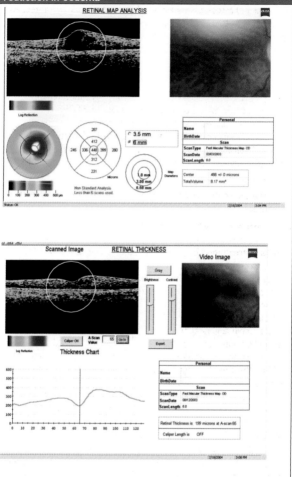

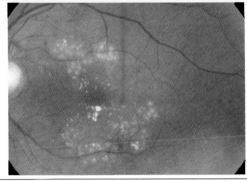

17.4.3 **Drugs given by intra-vitreal or subtenons routes**

Intra-vitreal injection of drugs has been shown to be an effective and safe means of drug delivery to the retina and is being used increasingly in cases of diffuse or ischaemic diabetic maculopathy, where laser treatment may not be effective. The procedure requires a sterile technique and must be done by an experienced ophthalmologist but can be given in a designated 'clean room' on an outpatient basis, in order to reduce to a very low risk of introducing serious infection into the vitreous cavity, resulting in endophthalmitis.

Triamcinolone was the first intra-vitreal drug to be used in large amounts and has been shown in a number of case series to be effective in reducing macular oedema. The main side effect is that as it is a steroid, there is a significant risk that intra-ocular pressure might become elevated although in most cases this is not a significant problem. In some cases, however, it can be, so this drug is probably contraindicated in cases with glaucoma. Cataract is also invariable 18 months later following repeated injection.

A number of anti-VEGF drugs have also been used by intra-vitreal injection (Figure 17.5) including bevacizumab, ranibizumab, and pegaptanib. These all work by inhibiting VEGF and as a result decrease vascular permeability of retinal vessels. At present, there are no licensed anti-VEGF drugs for diabetic retinopathy available but they are either used off-label, in the case of bevacizumab (Avastin®) and triamcinolone (Kenalog®), or are being used in clinical trials.

Figure 17.5 Intra-vitreal injection technique

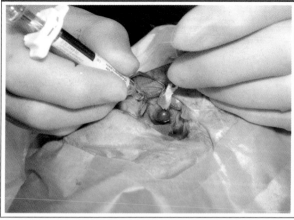

Intra-vitreal delivery of all the above drugs yields a fast action time with reduction of the retinal thickness and visual improvement being detected within a few hours of injection. The disadvantage, however, is that this effect wears off within a few weeks or months and requires repeat injection. As a result of this, combination of the drugs with conventional laser treatment may provide the best long-term treatment.

Triamcinolone can also be given as a peri-ocular injection into the subtenons space which is theoretically safer than the intravitreal route as the globe of the eye is not entered and is used for the administration of a depot of drug which is slowly absorbed into the retina through the sclera. The effect of such injections may last for several months.

The drawback is that the result of subtenons injection is less predictable than intra-vitreal injection and there may be difficulty in some patients in preventing reflux of the drug. There is also the risk of a prolonged rise in intra-ocular pressure in susceptible cases.

17.5 **Surgery for advanced DR**

Pars plana vitrectomy is a specialized procedure which is the domain of highly specialist-trained ophthalmic surgeons. Vitrectomy surgery is used to achieve specific goals, which may limit or halt the progress of advanced diabetic eye disease. These are as follows:

• To remove vitreous opacity (commonly vitreous haemorrhage, also intra-ocular fibrin, or cells) and/or fibrovascular proliferation (severe extensive proliferative retinopathy; anterior hyaloidal fibrovascular proliferation) (Figure 17.6)

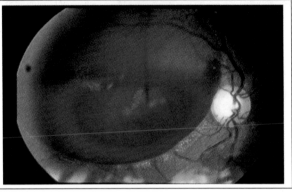

Figure 17.6 Large pre-retinal haemorrhage in patient with PDR. Repeated haemorrhages required vitrectomy to be performed

- To allow completion of pan-retinal laser photocoagulation (with the endolaser, introduced into the vitreous cavity or with the indirect laser ophthalmoscope), or direct ciliary body laser photocoagulation
- To relieve retinal traction, tractional displacement or ectopia, or traction detachment by removal or dissection of epiretinal membranes, in cases of non-rhegmatogenous retinal detachment
- To achieve retinal reattachment by closure of breaks and placement of internal tamponade (in cases of combined traction/rhegmatogenous detachments)
- To remove the posterior hyaloid face in some cases of diffuse macular oedema with posterior hyaloid face thickening.

Vitrectomy surgery now allows many cases of advanced retinopathy to be salvaged with resultant retention of vision. Surgery can be performed under local anaesthesia as a day case, but in prolonged procedures general anaesthesia may be preferable.

17.6 Cataract surgery in diabetic patients

Patients with diabetes are more likely to develop cataract at an earlier age and it is more likely to progress quicker than in the normal population. If fundus visualization or photography is difficult, cataract surgery is indicated to visualize the retina and apply laser treatment if indicated.

Small incision phacoemulsification with a foldable lens implant is the preferred current option and surgery is performed as a day case with local anaesthesia. Generally if laser treatment is required it is best to perform this prior to cataract surgery if possible, but if visualization of the fundus is difficult due to cataract, laser treatment can be applied intra-operatively with the indirect ophthalmoscope mounted laser or a few days later.

Post-operative review is critical and in cases with severe retinopathy early review is essential.

Further reading

Al-Hussainy S, Dodson PM, Gibson JM (2007). Pain response and follow up of patients undergoing pan-retinal laser photocoagulation with reduced exposure times. *Eye* (advance online publication 2008).

Bloom SM and Brucker AJ (1997). *Laser surgery of the posterior segment.* Lippincott-Raven, New York.

DRS Research Group (1981). Photocoagulation treatment of proliferative diabetic retinopathy: Clinical applications of Diabetic Retinopathy Study findings, DRS report number 8. *Ophthalmology*, **88**: 583–600.

ETDRS Research Group (1985). Photocoagulation for diabetic macular edema: Early Treatment Diabetic Retinopathy Study Report Number 1. *Archives of Ophthalmology*, **103**:1796–806.

Hee MR, Puliafito CA, Wong C, Duker JS, et al. (1995). Quantitative assessment of macular edema with optical coherence tomography. *Archives of Ophthalmology*, **113**:1019–29.

Jonas JB, Kreissig I, Sofker A, Degenring RF (2003). Intravitreal injection of triamcinolone acetonide for diabetic macular edema. *Archives of Ophthalmology*, 121: 57–61.

Olk RJ (1986). Modified grid argon (blue green) laser photocoagulation for diffuse diabetic macular edema. *Ophthalmology*, **93**: 938–50.

Royal College of Ophthalmologists (2005). Guidelines for diabetic retinopathy, at www.rcophth.ac.uk.

Screening intervals, other DR grading systems and visual acuity scales

Screening intervals

Population studies suggest that diabetic subjects without any diabetic retinopathy (DR) are unlikely to develop sight-threatening retinopathy within 2 to 4 years, but these were in white Caucasian populations only. The Liverpool eye study is one of the largest surveys of the incidence of DR in both type 1 and 2 diabetic subjects. The conclusion for type 1 diabetes was that 2–3 yearly intervals for those patients without retinopathy was feasible because of the low risk of progression to sight-threatening forms. For type 2 diabetes, the conclusion was for a 3-year interval in those with no retinopathy changes. In addition, a US modelled outcomes and costings for eight strategies including routine screening every 2 to 4 years and re-screening for those with retinopathy at 6-month to 2-year intervals produce benefits which outweighed the costs. In contrast one- and two-year intervals have been compared in Iceland and although a 2-yearly interval was sufficient for people without retinopathy, it led to more practical problems than annual screening.

It is therefore not the scientific issues that have been persuasive, but rather the practical issues. For diabetic patients, an annual medical review is standard and therefore an annual retinopathy check fits with this concept. This is supported by a consensus amongst experts in Europe that yearly screening is appropriate, and the UK national screening model has endorsed this, at least initially.

DR grading systems; the four nations of the United Kingdom, Europe, and the United States

The primary aim of the National Screening programme for DR in the United Kingdom is to detect diabetic eye disease at a stage at which visual loss can be limited by laser and other treatments. A working party for England and Wales was convened and reported the minimum dataset of retinopathy grades into four levels (R and M grades) in 2003, as described in Chapter 11. In the Scottish scheme there is considerable overlap, but major differences are apparent: the use of a single macula-centred image, the avoidance of routine mydriasis, and the inclusion of a more complex grading protocol.

Figure A1 The American Academy of Ophthamology Diabetic Retinopathy Staging (2002)

Diabetic Retinopathy (DR)
American Academy of Ophthalmology (AAO) Staging Guideline

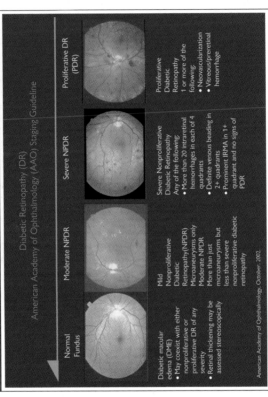

Normal Fundus	Moderate NPDR	Severe NPDR	Proliferative DR (PDR)
Diabetic macular edema (DME) • May coexist with either nonproliferative or proliferative DR of any severity • Retinal thickening may be assessed stereoscopically	Mild Nonproliferative Diabetic Retinopathy(NPDR) Microaneurysms only Moderate NPDR More than just microaneurysms but less than severe nonproliferative diabetic retinopathy	Severe Nonproliferative Diabetic Retinopathy Any of the following: • More than 20 intraretinal hemorrhages in each of 4 quadrants • Definite venous beading in 2+ quadrants • Prominent IRMA in 1+ quadrant and no signs of PDR	Proliferative Diabetic Retinopathy 1 or more of the following: • Neovascularization • Vitreous/preretinal hemorrhage

American Academy of Ophthalmology, October, 2002.

The grading system, suggested by the American Academy of Ophthalmology for the United States, is based on the Early Treatment of Diabetic Retinopathy Study (ETDRS) using seven field stereoscopic retinal photography. This grading system is used in research studies and has levels of 10 through to 85, termed mild non-proliferative (levels 10–35), moderate to severe non-proliferative (levels 43–53), high risk proliferative to advanced proliferative DR (levels 61–85); see Figure A1. This system has been considered complicated for routine clinical use, the United Kingdom have continued with the classification of background, pre-proliferative, proliferative and maculopathy.

The National Screening Committee (NSC) recommended that to define maculopathy, the distance of the lesion from the fovea is critical, that is, any exudate within 1 disc diameter (DD) of the centre of the fovea is significant. The definition is based on the best predictors of macula oedema, thereby the best surrogate markers on two-dimensional (2D) photographs (see Chapter 11). There are additions to the maculopathy grading, based on local variations and protocols. Some schemes use subdivisions of maculopathy to M1a and M1b. The Birmingham scheme uses the term maculopathy non-referable (MNR) to describe the presence of haemorrhages or microaneurysms within 1DD of the centre of the fovea but with visual acuity (VA) of 6/9 or better (shown in Figure A2).

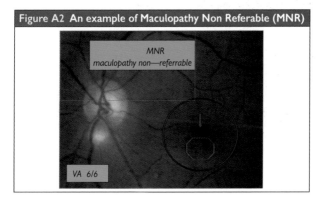

Figure A2 An example of Maculopathy Non Referable (MNR)

MNR
maculopathy non—referrable

VA 6/6

Of importance to treatment of maculopathy, the ETDRS study observed benefit in those that it defined as having 'clinically significant macula oedema' (CSMO). The definitions are complicated but the essence is the presence of exudates and retinal thickening at or within 500 microns of the macula centre (i.e. fovea), or 1 disc area of retinal thickening within 1DD of the macula centre (Chapter 17).

Visual Acuity Scales (VA)

The VA scale described in Chapter 10 uses the Snellen and Logmar charts. There are differences across the globe in visual scales used with the Snellen—feet, Snellen—metre, Decimal, and Logmar recordings. In particular, the research studies use either logmar or the decimal method, and Snellen—feet is used in clinical practice in the United States. Table A1 shows the methods and comparable VA scores.

Table A1 The comparative values of VA on the different scales used across Europe and the United States			
Snellen—Feet	Snellen—Metres	Decimal	Logmar
20/200	6/60	0.10	1.00
20/160	6/48	0.13	0.90
20/120	6/36	0.17	0.78
20/100	6/30	0.20	0.70
20/80	6/24	0.25	0.60
20/60	6/18	0.33	0.48
20/50	6/15	0.40	0.40
20/40	6/12	0.50	0.30
20/30	6/9	0.63	0.18
20/25	6/7.5	0.80	0.10
20/20	6/6	1.00	0.00
20/16	6/4.8	1.25	−0.10
20/12	6/3.6	1.67	−0.22
20/10	6/3	2.00	−0.30

Index

A

accreditation of competence 148
ACE inhibitors 152–4
acquired pigmented lesions 81–2
Acquired Prior Experiential Learning (APEL) 149
Actrapid® 8
adequate view images 109–10
administration of screening programmes 127, 132
annual reports 130
exclusions from screening 130–2
patient list 127–9
advanced diabetic eye disease 71–2
gliosis 74–5
National Screening Programme 78
rubeosis iridis 77
rubeotic glaucoma 77
subhyaloid/pre-retinal haemorrhages 72–3
tractional retinal detachment 76–7
vitreous haemorrhage 73–4
advanced glycosylation end products (AGEs) 158–9
age factors
consent for screening 131
diabetes mellitus 4
diabetic retinopathy 41
screening 41, 116, 130, 131
age-related macular degeneration (AMD) 23
drusen 79
treatment 157
alcohol moderation 7
aldose reductase inhibitors 156
American Academy of Ophthalmology 173–5
aminoguanidine 159
angiotensin receptor blockers (ARBs) 152–4, 156
annual reporting for screening programmes 130
anterior chamber anatomy
photography 98
anterior chamber angle, anatomy 18

anterior segment of the eye, anatomy 18–20
anti-oxidants 159
anti-VEGF drugs 168–9
Apidra® 8
aqueous humour 19–20
arbitration graders 119, 120
argon lasers 162, 163
arteriosclerotic disease 88
aspirin 8, 151, 155, 156, 159
asteroides hyalosis 91, 92
photography problems 100, 102
atorvastatin 155
Avastin® 168
axons, retina 21

B

background diabetic retinopathy 45, 59
cotton wool spots 47–8
exudation 47
grading 107, 175
haemorrhages 46
maculopathy 49
microaneurysms 45–6
bear track pigmentation of retina 81
bevacizumab 168
blindness see visual loss and blindness
blind spot 24
blood pressure control 152, 154, 156
blot haemorrhages
background diabetic retinopathy 46
pre-proliferative retinopathy 61
branch retinal vein occlusion (BRVO) 85–6
browning effect 5
Bruch's membrane 23, 79

C

calcium channel blockers 152
call/recall system 129
Canal of Schlemm 20
candesartan 153
carotid artery disease 90
carotic artery endartectomy 88
cataracts 6, 34–5
photography problems 100, 111

surgery 170–1
triamcinolone contraindicated 168
central processing units (CPUs) 137
central retinal vein occlusion (CRVO) 87, 88
cerebrovascular disease 6
Certificate in Diabetic Retinopathy Screening 148–9
children
diabetic retinopathy epidemiology 41
diabetic retinopathy screening 116, 130
consent issues 131
cholesterol serum
diabetic retinopathy 43
lipid-lowering therapy 155
cholesterol embolus 88
choriocapillaries 22, 23
choroid 23
malignant melanoma 82
choroidal infection 84–5
choroidal naevi 81, 82
choroiditis 85
ciliary body 19
ciliary muscle 19
circinate exudation, diabetic maculopathy 54, 55
circle photographic artefact 100, 101
classification of diabetes mellitus 4
type 1 diabetes 4
type 2 diabetes 4–5
client computers 135
clinically significant macula oedema (CSMO)
definition 175
treatment 55, 165
communication
by ophthalmologists 162
by screeners 118
of screening results 118
complications of diabetes 5
macrovascular disease 5, 6
microvascular disease 5, 6
compression of images 139, 140–3
computer, anatomy of a 135
cone cells 22, 23, 50
congenital hypertrophy of the retinal pigment epithelium (CHRPE) 81

congenital pigmentation of the retina 81
consent for screening 131
contraceptive pill 48
cornea 18, 19
corticol cataracts 35
cosine transform 140
cotton wool spots
  background diabetic retinopathy 47–8
  branch retinal vein occlusion 86
  pre-proliferative retinopathy 60–1
cranial nerve palsies 37–8
cystoid maculopathy 57, 58
cytomegalovirus 84

D

dark photos 100
data collection 143–5
data transfer 145
detemir 8
Diabetes Competence Framework 147
diabetes mellitus 1–2
  classification 4–5
  complications 5–6
  definition 3–4
  diagnostic pathway 3
  ocular complications 33–4
    cataracts see cataracts
    cranial nerve palsies 37–8
    diabetic maculopathy see diabetic maculopathy
    diabetic retinopathy see diabetic retinopathy
    glaucoma see glaucoma
  principles of treatment 6–8
diabetic maculopathy 49, 58
  anatomical features of the macula 22, 23, 50
  classification 52–8
  development 50–1
  epidemiology 40, 41, 42
  exudation 47
  grading (M grade) 108
  screening 51
  treatment 165–9
  visual loss 12
diabetic microangiopathy 38
diabetic nephropathy 44
diabetic retinopathy (DR) 6, 38–40
  epidemiology and risk factors 40–4
  ophthalmology care, patients already in 132
  retinopathy grading (R grade) 107, 108
  visual loss 40, 151

see also advanced diabetic eye disease; background diabetic retinopathy; pre-proliferative retinopathy; proliferative retinopathy; screening; treatment, diabetic retinopathy
diagnostic pathway of diabetes mellitus 3
diet 5, 7, 8
diffuse maculopathy 54, 55, 56, 58
digital retinal photography
  acceptable images
    NSC standards/targets 103
    taking 98–9
  cotton wool spots 47
  information technology 138–43
  manipulation of images 111–2
  non-grading photographers 107
  problems 100–2
  quality of images 98–9, 109–11
  reflection and glare 26, 29–30
    cotton wool spots, differentiation from 47
    exudation, differentiation from 47
    pseudophakia 30, 31
diode laser technology 162
diplopia 37
directly connected data collection 144–5
Disability Discrimination Act 131
dot haemorrhages see blot haemorrhages
double vision 37
drop instillation using mydriasis 96
  contraindications 96–7
drusen, retinal 23, 79–80
duration of diabetes, and risk of retinopathy 40, 41, 43

E

early maculopathy 52, 53
education see training in retinal screening
emboli, retinal arteriolar 88
energy metabolism 1, 2
England, grading system 173
epidemiology of diabetic retinopathy 40–2
  risk factors 42–4
epithelial cells 22
ethnic factors

diabetes mellitus 4
  diabetic retinopathy 40
  retinal pigmentation 26, 27
exclusions from screening programme 130–2
external limiting membrane, retina 21
exudation
  background diabetic retinopathy 47
  diabetic maculopathy 51, 52, 53–6, 58
  and drusen, differentiation between 79, 80
  red-free image manipulation 111
eye
  anatomy 17–18
    anterior segment 18–20
    fundus 24–32
    posterior segment 20–4, 50
  problems see diabetes mellitus, ocular complications

F

fenofibrate 151, 155
fibrates 154–5, 159
financial issues
  screening programme 14
  visual loss, costs of 14
fixed location screening services 116
fluorescein angiography (FFA)
  branch retinal vein occlusion 86
  central retinal vein occlusion 87
  diabetic maculopathy 165, 166
focal maculopathy 54, 55, 56, 58
fovea
  anatomy 22, 23, 50
  appearance 26
  glare in digital photography 30
foveal burn 164–5
foveal reflex 30
fundus
  appearance (healthy) 24–5
  normal variations 26–32
  ophthalmic lesions 79
    inflammatory disease 84–5
    pigmentation abnormalities 81–4
    rarer abnormalities 91–3
    retinal drusen 79–80
    retinovascular disorders 85–90

G

ganglion cells, retina 21
gender factors, diabetes
    mellitus 4
genetic factors, diabetic
    retinopathy 43–4
glare, digital retinal photog-
    raphy 26, 29–30
    cotton wool spots,
        differentiation from 47
    exudation, differentiation
        from 47
    pseudophakia 30, 31
Glargine® 8
glaucoma 37
    iris neovascularization 37,
        64
    primary open-angle 37
    and pupil dilatation 96–7
    rubeotic 37, 77
    triamcinolone contraindi-
        cated in 168
gliosis 74–5
glitazone 7
glucose 1–2
    browning effect 5
    definition of diabetes 3
    intolerance 3, 4
    principles of diabetes
        treatment 6–7
    tolerance test 3
glycaemic control 152, 153,
    154, 156
glycated haemoglobin
    (HbA1c) 5, 152
good view images 109, 110
graders 119
    grading pathways 119–20
    job role 105–7
grading 105
    environment 105, 106
    image manipulation
        111–2
    image quality 109–11
    laser, presence of 109
    maculopathy (M grade)
        108
    national differences
        173–5
    National Minimum
        Grading Standards 107
    patient outcomes from
        108
    retinopathy (R grade) 107,
        108
    step-by-step guide 113
growth hormone
    antagonism 157

H

haemoglobin, glycated
    (HbA1c) 5, 152
haemorrhages
    and aspirin 155

background diabetic
    retinopathy 46
    branch retinal vein
        occlusion 86
    early maculopathy 52
    pre-proliferative
        retinopathy 61
    retinal 155
    subhyaloid 72–3
    vitreous see vitreous
        haemorrhage
hard disc drive 137
hemi-central retinal vein
    occlusion (hemi-CRVO)
    87
herpes virus infections 84
Hollenhorst plaque 88
Humalog® 8
hyperglycaemia
    cataracts 34
    diabetic maculopathy 50
    diabetic retinopathy
        38–40
    gene expression 44
hyperlipidaemia
    diabetic retinopathy 43
    retinovascular disease 35
hypertension
    control 152, 154, 156
    cotton wool spots 48
    macroaneurysms 90
    retinovascular disease 35
    visual loss 12
hypertensive retinopathy
    88–9
hypoglycaemia 7

I

images
    compression 139, 140–3
    information technology
        138–43
    jpeg 140
    manipulation 111–2
    NSC standards/targets
        103
    problems 100–2
    quality 98–9, 109–11
    size 141–3
    taking acceptable 98–9
    see also digital retinal
        photography
impaired fasting glucose 3, 4
impaired glucose tolerance
    3, 4
incretins 7, 8
indirect remote data collec-
    tion 144
inferior arcade 25
inflammatory disease 84–5
information technology (IT)
    133–5, 145
    anatomy of a personal
        computer 135
    bits and bytes 135–6

central processing units
    137
    hard drive storage 137
    images 138–9
        compression 139, 140–3
        jpeg 140
        size 141–3
    memory 136
    operating system 138
    screening models 143–5
    software 138
informed consent for
    screening 131
inner nuclear layer, retina
    21
inner plexiform layer, retina
    21
insulin 2, 152
    deficiency 2
    principles of diabetes
        treatment 7, 8
    replacement therapy 5
        prevalence of retinopa-
            thy 42
        risk factors for retinopa-
            thy 44
    resistance 2, 5
    type 1 diabetes 4
    type 2 diabetes 4
internal limiting membrane,
    retina 21
intra-retinal microvascular
    abnormalities (IRMAs)
    62
intra-vitreal injection of
    drugs 168–9
iris 19
iris clip lens 97
iris neovascularization
    (iris rubeosis)
    advanced diabetic eye
        disease 77
    glaucoma 37, 64
    proliferative retinopathy
        64, 68
ischaemic maculopathy 12,
    51, 52, 56, 57, 58
ischaemic optic neuropathy
    36
Isophane® 8

J

jpeg images 140

K

kenalog® 168

L

lacquer cracks 83
laser treatment 162–3
    diabetic maculopathy 165,
        166, 168, 169

grading 109
macroaneurysms 90
proliferative retinopathy
163–5
scars 81, 84
side effects 164–5
lens (camera) artefacts 101, 102
lens (eye) anatomy 18, 19, 20
lipid disorders 12
lipid levels
diabetic retinopathy 43
hyperlipidaemia 35, 43
lipid-lowering therapy
154–5, 156
lisinopril 153
Liverpool declaration 14
Logmar chart 94, 175–6
lossless compression 139
lossy compression 139, 140

M

macroaneurysms, retinal
arteriolar 90, 91
macrovascular disease 5, 6
macula
anatomy 22, 23, 50
appearance (healthy) 26
branch retinal vein
occlusion 86
imaging methods 165–6
myopic crescent 31–2
see also diabetic
maculopathy
macula-centred view of
fundus 24–6
reflection and glare in
digital photography 30
maculopathy see diabetic
maculopathy
maculopathy grading (M
grade) 108, 113, 175
laser treatment 109
maculopathy non-referable
(MNR) 175
malignant melanoma of the
choroid 82
management see treatment
Masters degree in diabetic
retinopathy screening
150
melanoma of the choroid
82
memory, computer 136
mentally disabled patients
131
metformin 8
metiglinides 7, 8
M grade 108, 113, 175
laser treatment 109
microaneurysms
background diabetic reti-
nopathy 45–6, 48
early maculopathy 52, 53

red-free image
manipulation 111
microangiopathy, diabetic
38
micropulse laser technology
162
microvascular disease 5, 6
mitochondrial diabetes 5
mixed screening services
116
mobile screening services
116, 117
information technology
143–4
multidisciplinary team
diabetes treatment 7
glycaemic control 152
multifactorial interventions
156
mydriasis 96
contraindications 96–7
myelinated nerve fibres 28,
82–3
myocardial infarction 6
myopia 83
myopic crescent 31–2, 83

N

N3 144, 145
nasal-centred view of fundus
25
reflection and glare in
digital photography 30
National Assistance Act 15
National Minimum Grading
Standards 107
National Occupational
Standards 147
National Screening
Committee (NSC)
advanced diabetic eye
disease 73, 78
definition of screening
14
diabetic maculopathy 51,
58
digital retinal photography
standards/targets 103
grading 175
experience and workload
of graders 106
National Minimum
Grading Standards
107
image compression 143
pre-proliferative
retinopathy 63–4
proliferative retinopathy
67–8
screening programme
annual reports 130
exclusions 130
standards 122–5
National Service Framework
(NSF) for Diabetes 115

training and accreditation
in screening 147
nephropathy, diabetic 44
neuro-sensory layer 22
new vessels elsewhere
(NVE)
advanced diabetic eye
disease 72
laser treatment 163, 164
proliferative retinopathy
64, 65–6
new vessels of the optic disc
(NVD)
advanced diabetic eye
disease 72
gliosis 75
laser treatment 163, 164
proliferative retinopathy
64, 65–7, 68
NHS network 144
night-time vision, reduction
in 165
non-enzymatic protein
glycation 158–9
non-grading photographers
107
non-ischaemic diabetic
maculopathy 12
nuclear cataracts 35
nursing homes, patients in
132

O

operating system (OS) 138
ophthalmic treatment
161–2
cataracts 170–1
diabetic maculopathy
165–9
laser treatment 162–3
proliferative retinopathy
163–5
surgery 169–71
ophthalmology care,
patients already in 132
optical coherence
tomography (OCT)
165, 166, 167
optical storage 145
optic disc 20, 24, 25
optic nerve
anatomy 24
ischaemic optic
neuropathy 36
optometry-based screening
services 116
oral contraceptive pill 48
ora serrata 20
orlistat 7, 8
outer limiting membrane,
retina 21
outer nuclear layer, retina
21
outer plexiform layer, retina
21

P

pan-retinal photocoagulation (PRP) 162, 163–4
  side effects 164–5
pars plana vitrectomy 169–70
PASCAL Photocoagulator 162
Patient Group Directive (PGD), pupil dilatation 97
patient list for screening 127–9
pegaptanib 168
pericytes 50
peripheral vascular disease 6
peripheral vision, loss of 165
permanently inactive patient list 129, 131
personal computers (PCs), anatomy 135
  see also information technology
phenylephrine 96
photocoagulation therapy see laser treatment
photography see digital retinal photography
photoreceptor cells 22
  cones 22, 23, 50
  rods 22
photoreceptor layer, retina 22
physically disabled patients 131
pigmentation, retinal abnormalities 81–4
  normal variations 26
pioglitazone 8
PKC enzyme inhibition 158
polypharmacy 156
posterior chamber of the eye, anatomy 18
posterior segment of the eye, anatomy 18, 20–4
pregnancy
  cotton wool spots 48
  diabetic retinopathy 43
  tortuous vessels 30
pre-proliferative retinopathy 59–60, 68
  characterization 63–4
  cotton wool spots 48
  multiple 60–1
  grading 107, 175
  intra-retinal microvascular abnormalities (IRMAs) 62
  multiple deep round blot haemorrhages 61
  venous abnormalities 63
pre-retinal haemorrhages 72–3

prevalence
  diabetic maculopathy 49
  diabetic retinopathy 40, 41
  type 1 diabetes 4
  type 2 diabetes 4
primary open-angle glaucoma (POAG) 37
prisons, patients in 132
private patients 132
proliferative retinopathy 59, 64, 68
  epidemiology 40, 41, 42
  grading 107, 175
  NSC guidelines 67–8
  pathogenesis 65
  retinal signs 65–7
  tractional retinal detachment 76
  treatment 163–5
  visual loss 12
protein kinase C (PKC) enzyme inhibition 158
pseudophakia 30, 31
pupil
  anatomy 19
  dilatation 96
  contraindications 96–7

Q

qualifications in retinopathy screening 149–50
quality assurance (QA), screening programmes 121–2

R

randomly accessed memory (RAM) 136
ranibizumab 168
red-free image manipulation 111–2
reflection, digital retinal photography 29–30
remote data collection 143–4
renal artery stenosis 6
renal failure 6
reporting for screening programmes 130
residential care, patients in 132
retina 20–2
  see also fundus
retinal angiogenesis 65
retinal arterial occlusions 87
retinal arteriolar emboli 88
retinal artery occlusion 36
retinal detachment 91
  tractional 76–7
retinal drusen 23, 79–80
retinal haemorrhage 155
retinal hypoxia 65

retinal photography see digital retinal photography
retinal pigment epithelium (RPE)
  anatomy 22
  congenital hypertrophy of the (CHRPE) 81
  cotton wool spots, differentiation from 47
  exudation, differentiation from 47
  normal variations 28–9
retinal vasculature
  anatomy 23–4
  appearance 25–6
retinal vein occlusion (RVO) 35, 36
retinitis 84
retinopathy see diabetic retinopathy
retinopathy grading (R grade) 107, 113
  laser treatment 109
retinovascular disease 35–7
retinovascular disorders
  branch retinal vein occlusion (BRVO) 85–6
  central retinal vein occlusion (CRVO) 87, 88
  hypertensive retinopathy 88–9
  macroaneurysms 90
  retinal arterial occlusions 87
  retinal arteriolar emboli 88
R grade 107, 113
  laser treatment 109
rim artefact 100, 101
rinomabant 8
risk factors for diabetic retinopathy 40, 42–4
rod cells 22
rubeosis iridis see iris neovascularization
rubeotic glaucoma 37
  advanced diabetic eye disease 77
Ruboxistaurin® 151, 156, 158

S

St Vincent declaration 14
sclera 18, 19
Scotland, grading system 173
screeners 118
screening 11, 93
  advanced diabetic eye disease 78
  appointment 118–9
  background 48
  definition 14–15
  diabetic maculopathy 51, 58

drop instillation using
mydriasis 96
information technology
133–5, 145
basic technologies 135–8
images 138–43
screening models 143–5
intervals 173–6
photography
NSC standards/targets
103
problems 100–2
taking acceptable images
98–9
pre-proliferative
retinopathy 64
programme 115, 122
administration 116,
127–32
annual reports 130
exclusions 130–2
models 116–7, 143–5
patient list 127–9
size 116
standards 127–32
proliferative retinopathy
68
pupil dilatation, contraindications to 96–7
quality assurance 121–2
results, communication of
118
training and accreditation
147–8
Certificate in Diabetic
Retinopathy
Screening 148–9
higher qualifications 150
visual acuity testing 93–6
visual loss, reduction of
13–14
who to screen? 116
see also grading
secondary diabetes 5
server computers 135
Skills for Health 147
smoking
cessation 7, 43
diabetic retinopathy 43
retinovascular disease 36
Snellen charts 93–4, 95,
175–6
software programs 138
solid state laser machines
162
somatostatin 157
statins 8, 151, 154–5, 156,
159
stroma 19
subcapsular cataracts 35
subhyaloid haemorrhages
72–3
subtenons injection of drugs
169
sulfonylureas 7, 8
superior arcade 25

surgery
advanced diabetic
retinopathy 169–70
cataracts 170–1
vitrectomy 42, 170–1
indications 74
syphilis 84, 85

T

temporarily inactive patient
list 129, 130
disabled patients 131
ophthalmology care,
patients in 132
terminally ill patients 131
terminal illness 131
tertiary graders 119
thiazide diuretics 152
thiazolidinediones 8
tigroid fundus 27–8
tokenization 139
tortuous vessels 30–1
toxocariasis 84
toxoplasmosis 84
trabecular network 18, 20
tracking exudates, diabetic
maculopathy 54
tractional retinal
detachment 76–7
training in retinal screening
147
accreditation of
competence 148
Certificate in Diabetic
Retinopathy Screening
148–9
higher qualifications 150
treatment
diabetes
principles 6–8
type 1: 4
type 2: 5
diabetic retinopathy 151,
158–9
clinical need 151
conventional risk factor
modification 152–5
multifactorial
interventions 156
new potential therapies
156–8
ophthalmic 161–71
triamcinolone 167, 168, 169
triglycerides
diabetic retinopathy 43
lipid-lowering therapy
154–5
tropicamide 96
tuberculosis 84
type 1 diabetes 4
complications 6
diabetic maculopathy 49
diabetic retinopathy
epidemiology 40, 41–2
screening intervals 173

glycaemic control 152
principles of treatment 7
visual loss
causes 12
reduction through
screening 13
type 2 diabetes 4–5
complications 6
ocular 34
diabetic maculopathy 49
diabetic retinopathy
epidemiology 40, 41–2
screening intervals 173
glycaemic control 152
lipid-lowering therapy
154, 155
principles of treatment 7
visual loss
causes 12
reduction through
screening 13

U

ungradable images 111
United States of America,
grading system 173–5
USB memory sticks 145
uveoscleral outflow path 20

V

vascular endothelial growth
factor (VEGF)
anti-VEGF drugs 168–9
proliferative retinopathy
65
venous abnormalities,
pre-proliferative
retinopathy 63
venous beading,
pre-proliferative
retinopathy 63
venous looping,
pre-proliferative
retinopathy 63
Virtual Private Networks
(VPNs) 144, 145
visual acuity (VA)
measuring 93–4
during screening 95–6
scales 175–6
visual loss and blindness 11
causes 12–13, 33
advanced diabetic eye
disease 71–2, 73, 76
diabetic maculopathy 49,
51, 54
diabetic retinopathy 40,
151
glaucoma 37
pre-proliferative
retinopathy 64
proliferative retinopathy
67–8

retinovascular disease 37
tractional retinal
    detachment 76
definition 15
and screening 13–14, 131
vitamin C 159
vitamin E 159
vitrectomy surgery 42,
    170–1
indications 74

vitreous haemorrhage
    advanced diabetic eye
        disease 73–4
    and aspirin 155
    new vessels of the optic
        disc 67
    as side effect of laser
        treatment 164
    visual loss 68, 73
vitreous humour 20

W

Wales, grading system 173
weight loss 7
wireless networks 144

Z

zonular fibres 19
zonule 19